You need to read this book

> "... I'm so scared of waking up every day, this is so much more than just a skin disease."
>
> *Raffifox on Reddit*

Cure your psoriasis

Start your journey to banish this disfiguring and depressing disease.

Say goodbye to meds, creams and long sleeves by following simple instructions.

Having suffered from psoriasis for 30 years, I now take no medication. Not a single painful joint and I can run, ride a bike and wear a swimming costume in public. The only cream I use these days is ... in my coffee.

Long pants ... always

In the ten years since I graduated from med school, my 'annoying' psoriasis gradually became life-threatening. It attacked my joints to the point that I moved like an old person. My knees were swollen balloons; aching, unbending and seemingly untreatable. I put on 30kg and became a virtual cripple – physically and emotionally.

I tried everything

Having my knees drained and injected with cortisone and a year or two on chemo left me nauseous and vomiting four days a week. Knee acupuncture with pulsed electric shocks down the needles followed. Then a year of aggressive hormone therapy, painfully injected into my backside twice weekly. In desperation, I finally tried injections of radioactive yttrium into my knees.

Accidentally, I tried diet

Fifteen years later I was working on a low carb, high fat diet therapy and noticed that my psoriasis was slowly clearing. I wondered why a diet that removed sugars, grains and sweet fruit helped my skin and joints? I had to find out.

My 30-year journey as a doctor and psoriasis victim has resulted in the answers I share in this book. Answers I'm passing on as simple strategies to help you say goodbye to your psoriasis.

Heal yourself

Your psoriasis is far more than an annoying, unsightly skin condition. It has tentacles reaching deep into your body, affecting your heart, blood, nails and joints. Unchecked, it can even shorten your life.

Commit now to fixing your gut. Stop swallowing the meds and spreading odious stuff on your skin. Now is your time to end the charade of hiding the effects of this disease and to deal directly with what causes it.

This book will show you how to say goodbye to your psoriasis!

Tame Your Psoriasis From Within

A science-based natural therapy

Dr Howard Rybko

1st Edition April 2015
Copyright © Dr Howard Rybko

All rights reserved

Also available as an ebook from major online stores

Cover designed by www.wimrheeder.com
Edited by Nicolette Bosman of Ebbeevee Editing Services

All errors are my own

The right of Dr Howard Rybko to be identified as the author of this work has been asserted. No part of this publication may be reproduced, stored or transmitted, in any form or by any means, without prior written permission of the author.

While this work is written with the best intentions for use by both patients and medical professionals, it does not constitute medical advice. The reader is advised to consult with their chosen health professionals before embarking on any significant dietary and/or lifestyle changes.

Contact the author:
4Horsemen@biohacks.guru
www.thefourhorsemenofpsoriasis.com

For my beloved wife Gail
and our kids Caitlin, Paige and Gabriel

Thanks to:
Simone L. for getting me fired up and
Dr Barry Shmeizer (Gastroenterologist) for listening patiently

Table of contents

INTRODUCTION

The Four Horsemen of psoriasis 11
What is psoriasis? 13
Leaky gut 14
Re-imagining your gut 16
Program outline 18

WHAT

★ **DIET: THE FIRST HORSEMAN** 22
    How the diet works 24
DIET: Preparation 26
    Preparing your kitchen 26
    Learn how to read labels 28
    Shopping and supermarket survival 30
    Document yourself 33
DIET: Detox 35
    Food and supplements 35
    Food Stoplight 37
    Vital supplements 39
    Food sense 44
        Bone broth soups 44
        Changing your habits 45
        Sugar cravings 46
        The nightshades 48

  The dairy problem.. 49
  The alcohol problem 53
  The gluten problem... 55
  Say No to soy.. 57
  Good nuts and bad nuts.. 58
  Go easy on these! 59
  Daily-use items to avoid!.. 60
 DIET: Maintenance 66

★ **STRESS: THE SECOND HORSEMAN** **68**
 The effects of stress.. 68
 Managing your relationship with stress 73
 Breathing control.. 75
 Mindful eating.. 80
 Control your self-talk.. 82
 Back to nature 87
 Nurture friendships and relationships...................................... 91
 Get hugged daily 92
 Meditate... 94
 Go on a low-info diet 96
 Eat dark chocolate 98
 Sweat!... 99
 Stress apps 102

★ **ACTIVITY: THE THIRD HORSEMAN**...**104**
 Your weekly activity plan...106
 Stand up!..107
 Seven activity tips...109
 Aerobic training..110
 Walking well 114
 Resistance training 116
 Routines you can do at home..117

Gym routines	119
Body balance	122
Stretching and flexibility	124
★ **SLEEP: THE FOURTH HORSEMAN**	**126**
Light	131
Melatonin	132
Getting back to sleep	135
Sleep apps	138
SKIN CARE	**141**
GlyMag: A skin care treatment	141
Glycerin – humble wonder	142
Magnesium oil	144
GlyMag: How-to	145
General skin and nail care advice	146
Fighting a flare-up	148

WHY

More about psoriasis	152
THE GUT	**156**
The gut explained	156
Leaky gut in more detail	158
Into the toilet bowl darkly	162
The actual surface area of the small intestine	163
The brain in the gut	164
★ **DIET: THE FIRST HORSEMAN**	**167**
More on reading nutrition facts labels	167
Why our modern diet is so bad	171

- Missing stuff 172
  - Omega-3 fats 172
  - Vitamin D 174
- Supplements 174
  - L-Glutamine 174
  - Flax seed oil 175
  - Vitamin D 175
  - Magnesium 176
  - Biotics: Pre-, pro- and post- 178
- Joint pain from your gut 182
- Milk: A2 vs. A1 182
- FODMAP 184
- Cereal grains 185
- Bisphenol A (BPA) 187
- Good phytate, bad phytate 188
- Why you shouldn't use sweeteners 190

★ **STRESS: THE SECOND HORSEMAN** 192
- Cortisol 193
- Oxytocin: The hugging hormone 195
- Automatic nervous system 196

★ **ACTIVITY: THE THIRD HORSEMAN** 200
- Exercise variations 200
- Myokines 202

★ **SLEEP: THE FOURTH HORSEMAN** 205
- Your sleep clock 205

RESOURCES

RECIPES **210**
    Gut healing recipes 210
        Gail's bone marrow soup 211
        Gail's whole chicken soup 212
        Paige's chocolate coconut treats 213
        Homemade sauerkraut 213
        Milk kefir 216
        Slippery Elm tea 218
        Kombucha 219

GUIDES **221**
    Green foods 221
    Orange foods 221
    Red foods 222
    Vegetable Stoplight 224
    Carbs in common nuts and seeds 226

CHARTS **227**
    Bristol Stool Chart 227

APPENDIX **230**
    References 230
    Readings 240
    About the author 241

Introduction

The Four Horsemen of psoriasis

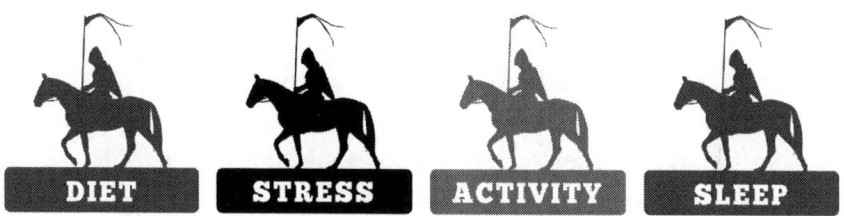

Tame these four wild horses to get better

I will show you how to work on the areas needed to restore your health and well-being and at the same time fix your psoriasis. I will provide clear strategies that will help you tame your psoriasis and make you whole and well again.

What affects your psoriasis?

Each horseman plays his part in your psoriasis. To properly heal yourself, you need to deal with each one. Together they contribute to the state of your gut, the dominant factor fueling your psoriasis.

1 – DIET

The food you eat contributes directly to the state of your gut. Eating sugar rich junk foods and grains worsens your gut and your psoriasis. Get your diet right, your gut will heal and in the process your skin will too.

2 – STRESS

Everyone knows that stress is bad for you. What is not so obvious are the effects of stress on your gut and immune system. Chronic stress raises cortisol levels, which damages your gut and wreaks havoc with your hormone balance. Once you lower your cortisol levels, your gut will heal, your weight will normalize, your energy levels will rise and so will your sex drive.

3 – ACTIVITY

Lack of exercise affects both your immune system and your gut. The effect on your health is so severe that the World Health Organization considers physical inactivity to be the fourth leading risk factor for global mortality.[1] Some light exercise will quickly enhance your immunity and boost important hormones.

4 – SLEEP

The amount of sleep you get and how regular it is makes a massive difference to your health. Lack of sleep directly affects your gut health.[2,3]

Your sleep habits and the amount of sunlight you get sets your body clock and dictates your body rhythms. Get your sleep patterns under control and your psoriasis will follow.

What is psoriasis?

Psoriasis is an autoimmune disease. Somehow, your immune system has become confused and is attacking you, damaging some of your cells and interfering with important bodily functions.

In common with almost all autoimmune diseases, psoriasis is accompanied by a damaged gut. This damage is called leaky gut (increased gut permeability) in concert with an imbalance in the types of bacteria that live in your gut (dysbiosis). A leaky gut is probably necessary for any autoimmune disease to develop, although other factors, such as genetics and your environment also contribute.

Along with your psoriasis, you may also suffer from:
- Digestive issues: Constipation or runny tummy (diarrhea), gas, bloating, Irritable Bowel Syndrome (IBS)
- Mental issues: Depression, anxiety or a sensation of a 'foggy' brain
- Chronic stress
- Sleeping difficulties
- Weight problems

You may also:
- Have been (or still are) on medication, especially antibiotics
- Spend most of the day sitting
- Seldom or never exercise
- Spend little time in the sun

Leaky gut

Leaky gut occurs when something foreign in your food makes 'holes' in your gut wall. These 'holes' allow an uncontrolled flow of partially digested food through your gut wall into your blood and body tissues. This spillover of foreign substances alerts your immune system, which then goes to work trying to remove the invaders. The immune system sometimes confuses these foreign substances with 'self' and starts to attack normal body tissue.

Everything we do in this program is aimed at restoring the health of your gut. A damaged gut is the spark that lights the fire of an autoimmune disease like psoriasis.

What affects your gut
- Stress levels
- Sunlight exposure affects your sleep patterns which, in turn, affect your gut
- Everything you eat and drink
- Things you rub into your skin
- Your activity levels. Sitting all day is bad for your gut.

What your gut affects
- Everything – your skin, your joints, your immunity, your brain and even your moods
- FYI: Fixing my gut fixed my joints and amazed my joint specialist, not that it stopped him from prescribing the $900 a month kidney killer meds to his other patients.

- Your gut even has a 'brain' of its own! Some scientists call it the 'second brain' and sometimes it can change your mind without you even realizing it.

Be better!

As your gut heals, you will steadily get better and will:
- Be leaner
- Fitter
- Sleep better
- Manage your stress better
- Probably even have better sex

Oh, yes! Your skin will get also better.

Re-imagining your gut

Since all our work is ultimately aimed at repairing and protecting your gut, you need to grasp one important concept before we kick off.

The inside of your gut is also outside your body

As unlikely as it sounds, your skin and gut are both totally exposed to the outside world. While your skin is obviously in contact with the outside world and all its dangers, it is less obvious that your gut is exposed in the same way.

The hole in the bagel pile

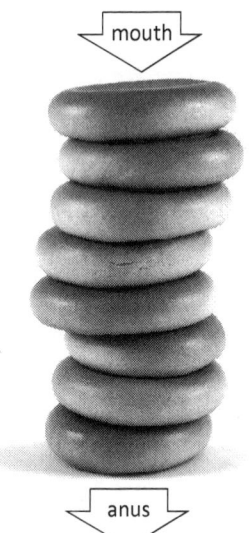

Try to picture yourself, arms at your side, standing next to a pile of bagels that is as tall as you are. The outside of the bagel pile is your skin. The hole in the middle is your gut.

Now stand on a chair and peep inside the hole in the bagel pile. You will see that the inside of the hole is just as exposed to the environment as the outside is. Just a little darker in there! The hole in the bagel pile is like the hole that runs from your mouth to the hole at the end of your gut – your anus.

Now try to imagine your gut as a long tube running from your mouth to your bottom, open to the outside environment.

Your skin

Your skin is the largest organ in the body. It protects your insides against a myriad of challenges, such as bacteria and viruses, liquids and fluids, oils, hot or cold surfaces, amongst other things. It also keeps things in. Damaged skin leaks both ways – in and out.

If you were to take the skin of an adult and lay it out like sheets of paper, the total area covered would be about two square meters (6.5 square feet).

Your gut

A big difference between your skin and your gut is the surface area they cover. Gut surface area is many times larger than your skin and is often compared to be the area of a tennis court. Recent research has, however, disputed the tennis court sizing and suggests that half a badminton court is more realistic. This is smaller, but is still a big area.[4]

Keep this in mind when next you are about to shovel some junk into your mouth.

Program outline

The program in this book is not hard to follow but it can and will show you brilliant results. All that is required is your commitment and some patience.

We need to deal with each of the four horsemen. We will deal with them in the order below but change the order if it suits you. After reading the information in this book you should ideally be able to make these principles a way of life.

This book has two sections: WHAT and WHY.

1. WHAT

This section tells you what you have to do, clearly and simply.

To benefit from the program, all you need to do is to read this section and put it into practice.

2. WHY

Read this section to understand the science behind the disease and its management. As you feel the need to know more, you can also dip into this section from time-to-time. It includes in-depth explanations of related concepts.

Much research and planning has gone into the development of this program and much of this is explained and expanded on in the Why section. I have tried to make the background and research as easy to comprehend as possible.

Terms we need to agree on

Poop

'Poop' in this book is a non-scientific way of saying: stool, feces, poo, solid waste, and so on.

Gut

'Gut' means your intestines, usually your small intestine, which is not actually that small. It is longer and thinner than the large intestine, measuring about seven meters (23 feet) in an adult. Depending on the context, gut can also mean your entire gut.

Bugs

When I refer to 'bugs', I mean bacteria. A bacterium is a single cell organism that lacks some advanced internal cell organs, such as a nucleus. They live in colonies and constitute the largest biomass on the planet. Bacteria flourish everywhere – in the deepest seabed, in the arctic, in radioactive waste and even in space craft. There are more bacteria in a single drop of gut fluid than there are people on earth.

The CORE of the program

Here is a bird's eye view of the core actions of the Four Horsemen program. Read each section in the book for more detailed information and instructions.

☆ DIET

You will never be hungry. You will also lose weight and have more energy. Your thinking will be clearer and sharper.

There are no portion size restrictions or weighing of food.

The foods you have to give up:
- Sugar
- Bread, potato, rice, pasta, grains, corn
- Sweet fruit
- Sodas including diet drinks

The foods you can have:
- Fats – natural and animal fats
- Alcohol

✯ STRESS

You will learn how to:
- Sleep better
- Breathe properly
- Eat mindfully
- Control your self-talk
- And more ...

✯ ACTIVITY

- Sit less
- Move your body

✯ SLEEP

Sleep eight hours a day

Skin care

Try the **GlyMag Skin Treatment** in the HOW section of this book. When used in concert with the four CORE actions, it can completely clear your skin. The GlyMag Skin Treatment uses the anti-psoriasis properties of two readily available, natural and safe compounds in a novel way that, with regular use, can restore normal skin.

WHAT

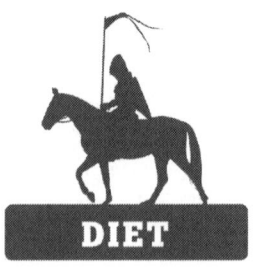

DIET: The First Horseman

It's easy to start an argument with your psoriasis doctor. Just say: 'Doc, I think that psoriasis begins in the gut.' Most traditional doctors will sit up straighter in their chairs and reflexively say, 'Nonsense!', or something similar.

Sadly, mainstream medicine today is focused on pushing meds. Why should there be a drive to find the real cause of your psoriasis, when a whole industry feeds off the sales of cures that patch up rather than heal?

I am not saying there is no place for traditional medical treatments for psoriasis. Of course there is. Rather, I think we should concentrate our efforts on fixing the cause of the psoriasis instead of medicating the results. It's a bit like painting over a wall that has damp in it. Eventually the damp will creep through and a new coat of paint will be required. To fix it effectively and completely, the source of the damp needs to be found and fixed.

So ... let's get fixing!

To fix your psoriasis, we need to work on the cause, the modern diet.

So you gotta diet

You can heal your psoriasis but you have to make changes to your diet.

If you don't have the determination to change your diet, then you are sadly wasting your time. You need commitment. Please be committed.

... and you gotta be patient

One of the joys of modern meds is the speed at which they work. It takes a day for a quick cortisone shot to dampen joint pain or to take the anger out of skin plaques. Even the creams work quickly (when they work!).

Doing things with diet takes time and patience. Please be patient.

... and you gotta be persistent

Persistence comes from commitment. I have already said you have to be committed. Dietary changes make a difference slowly, so you are going to have to be consistent. A time will come when your psoriasis calms down and you will have the luxury of cheating on your diet. Just not in the beginning, please!

The changes we are going to make to your diet must be followed for at least two to three months to make a difference to your health. You will get better. Be patient and allow time for your skin and joints to heal.

So here it is in a single sentence ... say it aloud a few times to convince yourself.

Doing things with diet takes time, commitment and patience.

I ... AM ... COMMITTED

How the diet works

What the diet does:
- It structures the food you eat
- It provides your gut with the right supplements so that it can heal itself

What the diet does NOT do:
- It does not limit portion sizes
- It does not ask you to weigh foods
- It does not expect you to count calories

The diet works In three phases
- Preparation
- Detox
- Maintenance

Preparation

In this phase, you decide on a start date. The programme provides an outline of the steps you should take to be prepared to start. A day or two of preparation will set you up to achieve the best results. Preparation outlines some practical steps to improve control over what you eat. It shows you how to remove temptations from your kitchen and how to shop smartly.

Detox

Detox outlines the steps you need to take to make sure that you eat healthy foods and avoid foods that damage your gut. Detox arms you with information to allow you to make better food choices.

Initially the diet modifications you will have to make are quite wide but, as your disease retreats, you can occasionally add some of your favorite foods. This makes the diet a lifestyle of eating well without it becoming a life sentence of abstinence from all the 'bad' foods that you enjoy.

Paleo and LCHF (low carb high fat/Banting) principles form the core of Detox and of the lifestyle that you will evolve.

This means that your diet restrictions are going to be:
- Sugars (carbs)
- Grains
- Dairy

Dairy restrictions will vary from person to person. Some people can handle dairy and this may allow inclusion of reasonable amounts of cream and butter without any ill effects.

Maintenance

You will hopefully make it through the easy days of Detox and find yourself looking at the Maintenance phase. This is the hard part! Normally quite a high percentage of my patients make it to Maintenance but many fall off the wagon as they slowly relax their grip on the lessons of Detox.

You can't relax but you can maintain if you remain vigilant and don't bend the rules too often. If you have successfully modified your gut biome during Detox, it becomes reasonably resilient to the occasional dietary transgressions.

DIET: PREPARATION

Before starting a new journey, it is always essential to prepare. On this journey, there are four simple steps:

1. Prepare your kitchen
2. Learn how to read labels
3. Shop for some 'getting started' basics
4. Document your starting point

Preparing your kitchen

One of the most important steps in preparation that you need to take is to ensure that your home is sugar and wheat safe. Do this by ridding your house of any foods, drinks or snacks that may trip you up in the early weeks of your new life.

Go through your kitchen, pantry, sweet cupboard and any other place where you stash snacks and remove any potential threats to your resolve.

This step acts both as insurance and as a symbol of commitment to your psoriasis and health goals.

You need to guard against occasional mood or hormone changes that will cause you to stray if the timing is right. If you happen to get home feeling miserable after a bad day, do you really need that chocolate bar, packet of sweets or tasty loaf of bread to be tempting you? It would be so much better if you had prepared for this by having the right food and snacks on hand to help you reach your goals.

Rid your kitchen of temptation. Go through this checklist and throw out (or give away) all the food items listed.

What to remove:

- Sodas, bottled and tinned drinks of any kind including diet drinks
- Fruit juice of any kind
- Flour of any kind – including whole wheat, buckwheat and other kinds of wheat
- Potatoes of any kind (sorry, but that includes sweet potatoes)
- Rice of any kind or color
- Sugar in all of its forms – including molasses, brown sugar and baking sugar
- Honey and syrups (honey is just liquid sugar)
- Artificial sweeteners – Xylitol and all similar types ending in '...ol' as well as any other sweeteners
- All 'lite' or diet-labeled foods – like lite yogurt or yogurt with fruit
- Any fruit except for the berry family
- Any sweets and chocolates including chewing gum
- Any foods with the word hydrogenated in the label
- Any vegetable oils – especially cooking oils and margarines

Finally, check all the food in your kitchen that comes in boxes. If it comes in a box it probably needs to go, so be sure to read the ingredient list carefully. If any have sugar, carbohydrate, glycemic carbs or have the word 'hydrogenated' in the contents, throw the stuff out!

If you see the word 'fructose' – throw.
If you see words like 'corn syrup' – throw.

Suggestion for those who share their kitchen with non-dieters

Make a special place for 'forbidden foods' and keep them there. Make sure that the non-dieters understand the reasons why you are keeping foods in a separate place. Make sure they know how important it is for you and try to get their cooperation.

The 'forbidden food' locker should be in a cupboard or a place that is discreetly out of sight and can be kept closed. The aim is to make it difficult for you to take food from the locker and to deter you in those momentary lapses of resolve.

Learn how to read labels

In order to succeed, you need to know your enemy. This enemy is **sugars** and **grains**, especially wheat.

Sugar hides everywhere

I use the word sugar and carbs or carbohydrate interchangeably. Sugar when digested turns into 50% glucose and 50% fructose. Some carbs are mixtures of glucose and other simple sugars.

Grains are a problem for psoriatics with leaky guts. There are many antigens in grains, including gluten (the main culprit) that can and will harm your gut membrane.

By avoiding sugar, you also avoid wheat and grains that are so bad for your gut. When it's digested:

- A slice of the finest whole-wheat bread turns into mostly sugar.
- A healthy apple is mostly sugar.
- A bowl of breakfast cereal turns to sugar.
- A supposedly healthy bowl of muesli often contains as much sugar as a cereal like Coco Pops.

The worst possible case is to discover that an item you are eating regularly is full of sugars and grains so is quietly sabotaging your efforts.

DIET: THE FIRST HORSEMAN

Net carbs (digestible carbs or glycemic carbs)

Ensure that you understand what Net Carbs are! This term refers to the digestible portion of carbohydrate in your serving and means the same thing as Digestible or Glycemic carbs.

The carbs in a food source are often made up of a digestible portion and fiber, which is not digestible. The number given for Total Carbohydrates includes both of these. In order to calculate the actual carbs that will affect your blood sugar, you need to know the Net Carb value.[5] Sometimes, but not always, the food label will tell you.

For example, a packet of wild brown rice sounds healthy, doesn't it?

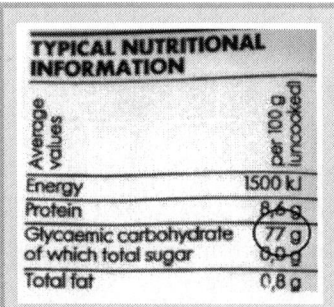

Sounds like something you can eat because it is low in sugar (0.4g)? Not! Look again at the label. It lists glycaemic carbohydrate at 77g. This is the business end of the stuff. Eat it and it will raise your blood sugar higher than the price of petrol.

Note that there is a scant 1.3g of fiber in the rice (72g minus 70.7g). So despite all the 'healthy for you' marketing blurb on the packet, this wild brown rice packs a potent sugar punch that will mess up your gut and make you fat in a jiffy.

Sugar alcohols

These are often added to low carb or 'lite' products to reduce the sugar content and the glycemic index. They mostly end in '...ol' – like xylitol, sorbitol, etc.

They are not a free meal and do count as carbs even though they will not raise your blood sugar sharply and thus stimulate insulin release. In general, they can be added in to your Net Carbs calculation at half their listed carb value.

Shopping and supermarket survival

Here is some advice on how to survive shopping in your supermarket. These tips on how to make the right choices can make or break the success of your Detox.

Supermarket isles are a minefield when you are shopping to avoid the hidden sugars and grains that are so deadly for your gut.

If you see it on TV, don't buy it!

An unbreakable rule is: Avoid any products you see advertised on TV. The more advertising a product gets, the surer you can be that it is not something you want to put in your body. The better the advertising, the poorer the quality of food.

Another important rule is: Avoid products that stress how healthy they are and those that proudly sport medically-based 'good for you' badges.

Your most important tool is your ability to read labels. So make sure that you have read and understood the principles of "How to read food labels" in the previous section.

Skipping aisles

One of my patients once said to me, 'You won't believe how many aisles I skip in the local supermarket.' One of these aisles should be the cereal aisle, because there are no cereals you can use on Detox.

Oils

Avoid all vegetable oils. Rather pick olive oils (cold-pressed extra virgin being the least refined and therefore the healthiest) or avocado or coconut oil for cooking with. A good tip for oils is to go for the darker varieties because, in general, the lighter the color of the oil, the more it has been processed.

Fats

Butter is good if you can tolerate a little dairy. The butyric acid in butter is especially good for your gut. Consider using some fermented butter as it contains vitamin K2 and is higher in butyric acid than normal butter.

I suggest eating a teaspoon of butter directly or in your food at least twice a day. Never use margarine, except for polishing your car tires. Avoid any product that lists hydrogenated fats and trans-fats as ingredients.

Sauces

Skip the sauces you find on supermarket shelves. Tomato sauce is a big suspect in this area as it is high in sugar and salt (skipping the tomato is also a good idea).

Also, most tomato sauce contains high fructose corn syrup. Check the labels of all salad dressings and other sauces carefully before dropping them into your trolley.

Sweets

There is unfortunately little you can buy in the sweet aisle. However, 85% dark chocolate makes for a good treat. The Lindt variety has just over 1g of carbs per block.

Nuts

Buy good unprocessed, unsalted nuts. They make excellent snacks and can be added to meals as fillers for breakfast as well as to salads. Remember: No peanuts, cashews or pistachios.

Fruit

Try to avoid fruit because most fruit today is enhanced and carries excessive amounts of sugar and fructose, which will feed the hungry sugar bugs in your gut. Fruit has a lot of fructose in it and this is the single most important sugar for you to avoid.

Good fruit to buy:
- Avocados: Buy lots of these and eat them as snacks or use as fillers for various dishes.
- Berries are also a good choice.
- An occasional apple is okay.

Dried fruit

Don't eat any dried fruit unless forced to do so at gun-point. As a rule of thumb most dried fruit is at least 50% sugar.

Fresh produce

Various greens are all good. Vegetables are good except for the few that are high in carbs, such as potato, sweet potato, beans, squash and lentils. Carrots and pumpkin can be eaten in small quantities.

Beans

It is best to avoid beans during Detox.

Meat and chicken

Where possible look for free range varieties or grass fed meats. Avoid low cost protein that has antibiotics and hormones in it.

Fish

There is quite a strong movement that says we should avoid all fish because of the mercury and heavy metal content. This may be true for fish from certain areas but it is hard to be sure. I recently tested a pescatarian patient who eats fish five days a week and his blood levels of heavy metals were low-normal.

However, I think that an occasional fish meal is probably good for you; sardines, salmon, and herring are good choices. Shrimp and scallops are good to eat and are also low in toxins and mercury.

Document yourself

It is always exciting to start a new life chapter. Before you rush off, take a few minutes to record where you started so that you can amaze yourself at your improvement.
- Weigh yourself and record your starting weight.
- Take some private pictures of yourself and any skin surfaces that you struggle with.

Food and poop diary

Write down the food you eat over a week.

It is also beneficial to note down your daily poop routine. You can do this in conjunction with the poop chart, which describes their appearance. I have included a Bristol Stool Chart in the Charts section to help you.

Charting will help you clarify:
- On how many of the past seven days did you poop?
- Were there any days where you pooped more than once?
- Were you constipated?
- Did you have diarrhea?
- Were you feeling bloated on some days?
- Did you have cramps?

If you had a day where you answered 'yes' to any of the above, then think carefully. Can you link a particular meal or even a specific food type to a gut issue above? If you think you can, purposely have the same food again and watch carefully to see if you develop any of the same symptoms. Use your detective skills and see if you can ferret out the food culprit.

A picture is worth a thousand words

On the left is a 'before' picture of my right calf taken in 2013 at a time when I was happy with my skin! Compare that to the picture on the right, taken in 2015. In the earlier pic I was still using a steroid ointment, which I no longer use. I find steroid creams redden the skin color and also make the skin more permeable to irritants.

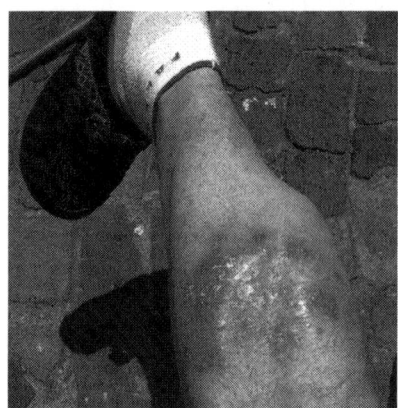 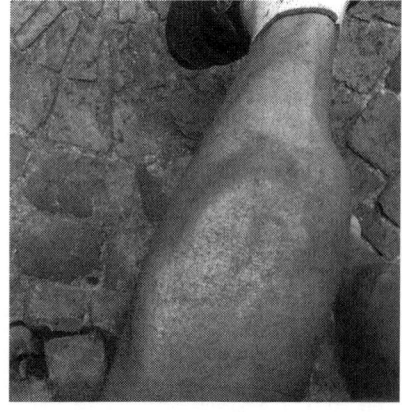

Blood tests (optional)

Lastly, here are a few optional blood tests you could have done:
- Vitamin D level (ideal level is between 50 ng/ml and 70 ng/ml)
- Waking cortisol level
- Waking glucose level
- Cholesterol panel (specifically note the triglyceride level)

DIET: DETOX

Food and supplements

The diet part of this program starts with Detox, which may take a few months or more. When you come out of Detox you can embark on an extended maintenance period which may last you the rest of your life. When you are on maintenance, you will be able to relax a bit and add back some of the foods prohibited during Detox.

It normally takes about four to eight weeks for Detox to kick in. Once it has, you will start to feel much better and the severity of your psoriasis will lessen progressively.

Detox is made up of two parts:
- FOOD: Changes to the food you eat.
- VITAL SUPPLEMENTS: The essential supporting supplements you need to take daily.

I know it's not easy to change your diet, and it's hard enough giving up all the stuff you love. Changing your daily habits makes this even harder. Well brace yourself; I'm going to make it a little harder still! You also need to add taking the Vital Supplements to your routine.

What will you have to give up?

Grains, corn and sweet stuff

Tasty healthy fats, some protein and lots of vegetables and leafy greens will replace your sugars and grains.

Despite its bad press, fat can be a wonderful thing. It makes you full quickly and keeps you full for much longer than a sugar-laced meal will. Fat also tastes good and it acts on the same happy center of your brain as sugar does.

Not so bad

It's not going to be so bad! After a few weeks you won't miss your bread, starch or sweet stuff. I have been working with patients and their diets for quite some time and I have learned that their main barrier is fear. Fear of loss. Let go of that fear and you will find that there was little to fear in the first place.

Aim of detox

Wheat and corn and most sweet things digest into simple sugars which are incredibly bad for your gut and for your psoriasis. Wheat and corn are also full of nasty antigens like gluten, which damage your gut lining. Dropping these foodstuffs from your diet will allow the inflammation in your body to subside.

Giving up these things will not be anywhere as hard as it sounds at first. The sugars you remove will be replaced by high fat, protein-based foods, along with tons of green veggies and some dairy if you can tolerate it.

Detox supplements

Remember to make sure you have shopped for the Vital Supplements that you will need to take daily.

Pooping properly

Detox will work best for you when you are pooping soft easy poop once or even twice a day. I also suggest the unthinkable: Look into your toilet every time you poop. What's in your toilet bowl speaks eloquently about the state of your gut.

What can you eat?

Below is an easy-to-scan list of what you can and can't eat. To make it easier to follow and remember, the list is arranged like the colors of a traffic light, dividing the foods into:

- **Green**: Allowed in quantity
- **Yellow**: Allowed in restricted quantities
- **Red**: Not allowed

Food Stoplight

Green

- Green vegetables
- Berries – all kinds
- Chicken with skin
- Meat with some fat
- Fish
- Eggs with the yolk
- Water (try for 5 glasses a day)
- Tea – all kinds

Orange

- Coffee (limited to 2 cups a day)
- Dairy (some cream in 2 cups of coffee a day and some cheese is permissible)
- Alcohol limited to 1 double tot of non-grain spirit, a glass of dry white or dry red wine or sherry – three times a week
- Artificial sweeteners in the smallest possible quantities

Red

- Cereal grains – wheat, barley, maize, rye, sorghum, millet, buckwheat, quinoa and oats
- Also grains such as spelt, emmer, durum
- Flour of any of the cereal grains
- Pasta
- Potato and sweet potato
- Rice (also a cereal grain)
- Anything marked low fat
- Milk (replace with cream)
- Fruit (all types except the berries)
- Juices – fruit and any kind whatsoever
- Sodas (all including diet varieties)
- Energy drinks and sports drinks
- Sports drink powders and bodybuilding supplements
- Sweets
- Ice cream (especially sorbet)

Vital supplements

Here are the vital supplements you need to take on a regular, daily basis to repair and protect your skin and gut:

1. Vitamin D3: 1,000–5,000IU
2. Magnesium (elemental): 200–400mg plus daily application of magnesium oil to your skin as part of GlyMag
3. Omega-3s: 1,000mg
4. L-Glutamine: 5–10g in water
5. Psyllium husks and/or slippery elm
6. Probiotics: As food or as an over-the-counter formulation

Aim to take these supplements every day. An occasional slip is fine but try your hardest to be consistent.

Vitamin D3

Take a vitamin D3 supplement that delivers between 1,000 and 5,000IU a day.

Do not take the vitamin D2 prescribed by many doctors! Vitamin D2 is ergocalciferol, a synthetic form of vitamin D made by exposing lichens, certain mushrooms and plants to high intensity ultraviolet light. Vitamin D3 is a much better choice than D2. D3 is cheaper, it does not require a doctor's prescription and it works almost twice as well as D2 in raising levels of active vitamin D.

Also, get into the sun! The sun is the best way for you get your vitamin D.

Magnesium

To treat psoriasis, I recommend two ways to raise and maintain magnesium levels. First, take a daily supplement that will deliver 200–400mg per day of elemental magnesium.

Second, rub magnesium oil onto your skin in the areas where you have psoriasis or into joints affected by psoriatic arthritis. Read more about GlyMag in the skin care section on page 141. Another way to increase your magnesium levels is to add a tablespoon of magnesium oxide or, if you can't find that, Epsom salts to your bath water.

Omega-3s

Raise your omega-3 levels with a supplement that will give you 1,000mg of omega-3s a day. You can use a good quality fish oil supplement or a tablespoon or two of organic quality flax seed oil. I take both – flax seed oil in the morning and two omega-3 capsules with my dinner.

L-Glutamine

Take at least 5g (a heaped teaspoon) mixed in water a day.

L-Glutamine comes in a powder form that is almost tasteless. It performs a healing action on the gut lining and can be taken more than once a day.

Psyllium husks and slippery elm

I recommend two insoluble fiber types: psyllium husks and slippery elm. They can be mixed and taken together or taken separately. You can get psyllium husks at most drug or health stores. Make sure the brand you buy is non-GMO.

Slippery elm may be a bit harder to find. Try some health stores or order it online. It can be taken on its own as a tasty tea. There is a recipe for it in the Recipe section.

The psyllium husks provide soluble fiber, which is fermented by the beneficial bacteria in your gut. The slippery elm also has healing properties, the most important of which is to sit on the surface of your gut lining, soothing and protecting it. The mixture of psyllium husks and Slipper Elm powder provided in the box below is ideal. However, if you can't get hold of both of them to make the mixture, start with one until your supplies come in.

Some of my patients complain about the psyllium husks. Not because of the taste of the psyllium, but rather because of the jelly-like consistency of it. Please don't let this put you off!

Drink the mixture in the morning or in the evening, whichever suits you best. If you are suffering from constipation, take it twice a day until you become regular again.

Some people have a sensitivity to psyllium husks, so start off with a small dose and then increase it to the standard dose below.

> **THE MIXTURE: Psyllium husks and Slippery Elm powder**
>
> Mix one heaped tablespoon of psyllium husks with a teaspoon of Slippery Elm powder in a glass of water. Use as much water as you are comfortable with.
>
> You can also take them separately. If you do so, it is best to have the Slippery Elm in the morning when you wake up and then the psyllium husks later in the day.

Probiotics

Probiotics are available in pill form or in a more natural form, as food. I am sure you would prefer to go the natural route which, as a range of fermented foods, is tastier and delivers better results.

Fermented foods

Eating fermented foods whenever you can is REALLY REALLY important. Remember that you must take a probiotic supplement when you can't get access to fermented food.

Refrigerators, pasteurization and the addition of vinegar to the foods in our supermarkets has increased shelf-life but at a cost. The price we pay is that all our food is dead when we eat it. Our ancestors, even as recently as our grandparents, ate a variety of fermented foods, which delivered a powerful health benefit as they supported both the growth of beneficial gut flora and the immune system.

Most of these foods were lacto-fermented. This term refers to a specific species of bacteria *Lactobacillus*. Numerous varieties of these cover us, our mouths, our gut and our surroundings.

Popular fermented food include:
- Sauerkraut (cabbage)
- Yogurt
- Pickles
- Kefir (milk)
- Lassi (yogurt)
- Kvass (rye)
- Natto (soybeans)
- Kombucha (tea)

There are many others in a diversity of cultures worldwide.

Live fermented – the solution

The most cost-effective and effective solution is to eat live bacteria in their natural environment. As an added benefit, you get to enjoy a tasty meal at the same time because live fermented foods deliver massive doses of beneficial bacteria. This is in contrast to probiotic supplements, which have to employ strategies to keep the bacteria alive until they finally make it off the shelf and into your gut.

Your own fermented foods

Try to make your own fermented foods. I have provided some examples in the Recipe section.

You can also look online for many examples and video demonstrations.

Off-the-shelf probiotics

Commercial probiotic supplements are available and packaged in a variety of ways. If you are not eating a variety of fermented dishes, remember to take a supplement. You can even do both.

How to choose a good probiotic

- Costs: Cheaper is seldom better
- Variety: Look for one that lists as many beneficial bacteria and strains as possible
- High counts: Look for high bacteria counts; quantities should be in the billions of bacteria per gram. Listed as CFU (Colony Forming Units), with bacteria counted either as single cells or as discrete clumps of cells.

Delivering probotics to your gut

This is more difficult than you would think. In the first place probiotic manufacturers have to keep the millions of tiny bacteria alive for extended periods of time. Manufacturers choose a variety of delivery methods, which affect the survival of your expensive probiotics. After all this, the probiotics still have to make it past the acid bath in your stomach.

The most effective and natural way to deliver large quantities of live probiotics to your gut is by eating them in your food. I have provided some easy-to-make food options in the recipe section of this book to get you started.

Food sense

Bone broth soups

If I could prescribe something that was critical to support your gut health efforts, I would insist once or twice a week that you have a delicious bowl of bone broth soup.

Bone broth soup has a number of important healing and protective properties. Bones and bone marrow have been part of our diet since time immemorial and for your gut health you must put these soups back on your menu.

Healing properties of bone broth soups include:
- Supports the immune system with a number of anti-inflammatory amino acids
- Reduces inflammation and joint pain (loaded with glucosamine and chondroitin)

- Gelatin in the broth holds liquids during digestion and promotes proper digestion
- Keeps bones strong with calcium and magnesium

Bone broth soups are made from cut up beef and other bones. It can also be made by cooking an entire chicken or a fish.

Bone quality

It is important to buy good quality bones. Ideally try to purchase organic and grass fed bones.

Changing your habits

You have to develop a bit of a siege mentality towards your food. Realize that swallowing bad stuff will later reflect in your skin and joints.

Don't be impulsive when shopping, when someone offers you food or when you order in a restaurant. Think before you chew as your split second choice has consequences.

Don't overeat!

- Listen to your body and eat only when you are hungry.
- Eat slowly and only as much of the permitted foods as you need.
- You don't need grains and sugar to survive! Humankind managed without them for two million years and so can you.

Don't eat too much protein

I encourage you to eat some protein, preferably good quality animal meat. Always mix the lean animal protein you eat with fat. The strategy of this diet is to replace sugars and carbohydrates with good quality fats.

This is NOT a high protein diet!

Your protein consumption should remain steady at around 1g per kg of body weight.

Do not pile your plate with chicken breasts or thick steaks as this unbalances the ratio of protein to fat. Piles of lean meat are not the way to go.

Aim to balance the quantity of protein you eat with at least an equal quantity of fat. Do this by adding fat such as the skin of the chicken, the fat of the meat or by adding whole eggs, avocado, olive oil or even bits of cheese.

Choosing carefully

Try to break the ingrained habit of always looking for low-fat foods. Remember this is a high fat program.

- Don't choose lean cuts when buying meat
- Eat the fatty bits when you eat protein
- Eat the chicken skin
- Don't pick the low-fat cheese or cottage cheese
- Don't buy or eat low-fat anything

Always choose high fat. Eating fat will make you feel full quickly. Never eat high fat and high sugar together. This diabolical combination raises insulin and drives any excess sugar and fat into fat storage (i.e. it makes you fat).

Sugar cravings

You may have sugar cravings during the initial weeks of Detox. This is normal, similar in some ways to giving up smoking or alcohol.

The great bug die-off

As you start Detox and drastically reduce your intake of grains and sugars, a profound change happens to the bug colonies in your gut. Remember that there are 10 times more bugs in your gut than cells in your body. Some bugs live on sugar, while others live on fiber. What now happens is that the sugar-eaters starve and die off.

Clear evidence shows that these sugar-loving bugs send chemicals to your brain that make you crave sweet foods. It sounds crazy but the bugs actually make you eat sweet foods so that you will feed them!

This is really important and should make you more determined to fight the craving. If you can last long enough, the bugs will die and your craving with them.

Fat strategy

Deal with these cravings most effectively by eating some fatty food, preferably mixed with some protein. Try some beef jerky, some cold meat, an avocado or even a handful of macadamia nuts. The fat in this type of snack quickly makes you feel full and will normally quench the craving. Avoid giving in and having a quick bite or two of something sweet at all costs.

Remember, besides the call of the bugs for more sugar, your cravings are part of a grain and carbohydrate addiction and you must not feed these cravings with sugar! Imagine if alcoholics were advised to have a little drink every time they felt the need.

Believe it or not, you will eventually lose your taste for sweet things, usually after a month or two. At this stage, you will be amazed to find that you can't eat the sweet stuff anymore, at least not in the same quantities you used to.

The nightshades

If you want to get better you are going to have to avoid eating nightshades, especially during Detox. Spoiler alert: If you love tomatoes, you're not going to like this! Your tomatoes must go.

The nightshades are a family of flowering plants that produce a range of alkaloid chemicals, some toxic to humans. Two of the best-known nightshade alkaloids are nicotine and capsaicin, the latter being the hot stuff in chilies and habaneros.

Belladonna

I'm sure the term 'deadly nightshade' must ring some bells? Nightshade is a poisonous plant also called belladonna because a small dose was used to make eye drops, which dilated (widened) the pupils of ladies' eyes, supposedly making them look prettier. Belladonna berries are small but pack a poison punch; it takes just two or three berries to kill an adult.

Potato – the world's favorite nightshade

The potato is the third largest food crop in the world and is eaten by over a billion people.[6] Because potato (not sweet potato) is also a nightshade, it contains some alkaloid traces.

Eating of potatoes has historically been associated with poor health. Heavy use was associated with dropsy, an old medical term for the swelling associated with heart failure.

Tomato – the world's second favorite nightshade

Tomatoes are growing in popularity and world production has increased year-on-year to reach 170 million tons in 2012.[7] Originally they were grown for display because of their bright red colors, and not as a food.

Many psoriasis sufferers eat a lot of tomato either whole or in sauces; I urge you not to and to avoid them completely during Detox.

Other popular nightshades

- Eggplants
- Tobacco
- Peppers, including bell peppers and chili peppers
- Red pepper seasonings – paprika, chili powder, cayenne, curry
- Pimentos
- Pepinos
- Goji berries
- Ground cherries (not fruit cherries)
- Ashwagandha

What this means for your psoriasis

There seems to be a consensus in both the medical and naturopathic worlds that eating nightshades is bad for psoriatics.

To repeat myself: Avoid eating nightshades if you want your psoriasis to heal. At the very least, I suggest that you avoid nightshades for at least the first three months of Detox.

The dairy problem

In the initial Detox period I prefer that dairy, in small quantities, remains part of your diet. It is such a versatile and tasty food group and can make Detox so much more enjoyable and sustainable. However, without realizing it, some people are sensitive to dairy. For these people, dairy must be omitted as well during the initial weeks of Detox.

Why initial? What sometimes happens is that as the gut heals and as its bacterial colonies shift toward normality, some sensitivities simply go away.

As an aside, I used to suffer from an almond allergy that was so strong that it once put me into a cardiac emergency theater. Staring up at the lights, I thought I was about to die. Since my gut has healed, I eat almonds every day with zero ill effects!

No milk

Milk is not part of this program and you must avoid it as far as possible.

Cream and butter are the main dairy products allowed as part of this program. Cheese must always be eaten with caution and certainly not in large quantities. A few slices in a salad or a single slice to nibble on are acceptable.

The two heads of dairy intolerance

It's not just a single substance in dairy that causes intolerance. There are two of them: casein, a protein; and lactose, a sugar. The easiest one to deal with is lactose intolerance.

Lactose intolerance

Lactose intolerance is common in adults. It is more common in Native Americans, South Americans, Asians and Africans as these populations had less exposure to milk products. People of European descent, however, normally tolerate dairy well because they have a long history of dairy use.

Intolerance of dairy occurs when there is a lack of a small intestine enzyme called lactase. Without lactase you can't break down the lactose sugars in milk. This leaves the tasty sugars for the bacteria in your small intestine. They eat these and cause gas, bloating and nausea in the process.

My patients often ask me how they were able to digest their mother's milk as babies but are now so lactose intolerant. What happens is that they lose the ability to make lactase when they are weaned and their exposure to milk stops.

Most people who are lactose intolerant already know it. Here are some signs that you are dairy sensitive. After eating dairy food you:
- have bloating and distension
- have stomach cramps
- can hear gas moving in your stomach
- develop a runny tummy, usually with diarrhea.

If you suffer from any of these symptoms, start your Detox without dairy. You can then add some dairy back, slowly and in small quantities, and see how you do.

Testing for lactose intolerance

A simple test involves the subject drinking water mixed with lactose sugar. Blood sugar levels are then checked at 30-minute intervals, watching for an upwards spike. This will indicate the digestion of the lactose sugar and its subsequent appearance in the blood. A variation tests the breath of the subject for hydrogen gas, caused as the bacteria digest the lactose.

This test can sometimes have dramatic consequences! When I was at medical school, we did a physiology practical that involved giving a subject a big glass of lactose. The idea was for us to graph the rise and fall in blood sugar levels over a three-hour period. Sadly Jonathan, the subject we chose, was totally lactose intolerant and within 30 minutes of starting the test his abdomen swelled alarmingly. We tried to calm him down but he ran from the lab and spent the rest of the afternoon in the toilets, cursing at anyone enquiring about his wellbeing.

Casein intolerance

A severe casein allergy will rapidly cause an allergic reaction resulting in swelling of the lips and body rashes. If severe, it may even cause breathing difficulties. This means that people with severe casein intolerance know it, and quickly too.

Casein intolerance is, however, a milder reaction that does not produce such dramatic signs but can do more long-term damage.

A1 and A2 casein

There is unfortunately another complication when it comes to milk.

Around 10,000 years ago, some say even longer, there was a split in the line of cows. Some cows produce milk containing A1 casein, while others produce milk with the A2 variety. Because of this, you can buy A2 milk in some countries, which you should buy preferably whenever you have the choice.

Some signs of casein intolerance
- Fever
- Mental changes – headaches, brain fog and general irritability
- Stiffness and aches
- Diarrhea
- Tingling in the hands and fingers
- Shortness of breath
- Chest pain
- Abdominal discomfort
- Abnormal hunger

Ways to reduce intolerance

Once your gut leakiness reduces, through using the methods in this book you might find that your milk sensitivity reduces. This is not wishful thinking. A recent study found that leaky gut caused by milk was reduced by a course of probiotics.[8]

Use A2 dairy products; this alone may reduce your intolerance.

You can also:
- Increase your vitamin D levels by taking higher doses of D3 (up to 5,000IU daily) and get some sun.
- Eat fermented foods whenever you can or take probiotics regularly.
- Add butter to your diet.
- Feed your gut flora with prebiotics. Prebiotics like inulin and resistant starch have been shown to increase butyrate production and reduce intestinal permeability (if you are not FODMAP sensitive).
- Get a handle on stress (or change how you approach it). Stress can increase intestinal permeability and disrupt your digestion.
- Exercise regularly. This can reduce stress-induced permeability.
- Watch your omega-6 intake and be sure to get your omega-3s. Omega-6 fats loosen tight junctions; the DHA in omega-3s has the opposite effect.

The alcohol problem

To drink or not to drink? That is the question.

This program explicitly allows for the careful consumption of alcohol.

Alcohol consumption has two problems for sufferers of autoimmune diseases:
- Alcohol increases intestinal permeability, which worsens the disease.
- Alcohol can contain glutens and other antigens that can worsen the disease.

So to keep drinking alcohol on this program, follow these rules:
- Always drink alcohol in moderation.
- Drink alcohol at most 3 or 4 times a week.
- Avoid grain-based alcohols completely during Detox (gluten containing).
- Mix drinks with water or ice only.

Prohibited alcohol includes:

- Most beers
- Most spirits
- Most cocktails

Allowed alcohol includes:

- Spirits: Grape-based vodka like Smirnoff Grape, Absolut Gräpe, Cîroc
- Spirits: Rum and tequila are okay, except when mixed with flavorings and coloring
- Beers: Many craft beers are made gluten free
- Dry wines can be used in moderation provided sugar levels are low

Grapes do not contain gluten, making wine a good choice for this program. There is some controversy about the wheat paste used by some winemakers for sealing the casks but most tests have shown the gluten content to be almost untraceable.[9]

Spirits of spirit

Most alcoholic beverages are grain-based and must be avoided. Also remember that the spirit of wheat and gluten lives in many distilled alcohols despite theoretically being removed by the distillation process. Distillers sometimes add back some grain-based mash after distillation. In other cases the spirit is not distilled enough times to remove the prolamins (gluten-containing proteins).

If you are cautious, you can still enjoy an occasional drink.

The gluten problem

Gluten is one of a number of foreign particles (antigens) that are part of the food we eat that produce an immune response in the gut. Gluten allergies are well studied and documented. In an allergic person, gluten causes cell damage or death to cells in the gut wall. This leads to leaky gut and its associated autoimmune issues.

Most tests for gluten sensitivity look for antibodies against alpha-gliadin, which is the most common, but by no means the only, protein fraction of gluten.

Gluten sensitivity is quite new

Over the last 50 years, gluten sensitivity has been increasing in world populations, causing it to become a major public health problem. A series of blood tests of airforce recruits, taken in 1950, was recently tested for gluten antibodies. These tests performed by Dr Joseph Murry of the Mayo Clinic showed that gluten sensitivity was rare among these 1950 airmen. Modern sensitivities are about 4.5 times higher.[10] I think this is because of greater exposure to wheat products combined with the genetic modifications in wheat that resulted in dwarf wheat pioneered by Norman Borlaug in the 70s and 80s.

Some signs that you may have a gluten allergy

- Poor digestion
- Headaches after eating
- Depression
- Anxiety or irritability
- Difficulty in focusing
- Brain fog

The graphic below shows how the long finger-like structures (villi) so necessary for absorption of food are stunted by gluten exposure in susceptible people. Damage to the villi that is this bad is called celiac disease (labeled Celiac Disease in the diagram).

Celiac disease

Also called gluten enteropathy, celiac disease affects the small intestine and is much more widespread than most people realize. It is estimated to occur in 1 in every 170 people worldwide.[11]

Gluten sensitivity is a much milder form of the disease and a lot more common than celiac disease. This means that gluten affects large numbers of any population that eat wheat, rye and barley even though it does not always show itself with obvious symptoms.

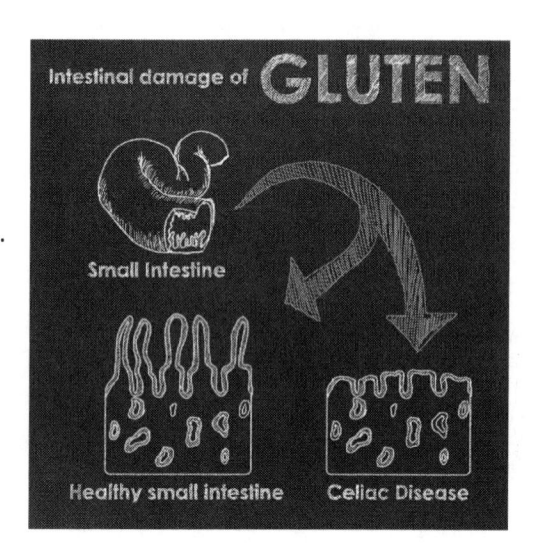

Avoiding gluten

Gluten is widespread along our food supply. Besides the obvious places such as wheat containing products, it can pop up in unexpected places. Some brands of instant coffee and flavored coffees, for example, contain some gluten. Be wary too of any food that says something like 'Gluten free but made in a factory that produces products containing gluten'. These kinds of foods often test for gluten, frequently in surprisingly high concentrations.

Say No to soy

It is best to avoid eating soy during Detox. Other than in its fermented non-GMO form, I suggest that you avoid soy completely.

Soy is good for your health in the same way that smoking is good for your lungs. When dealing with a leaky gut, it is best to avoid all soy products such as:
- Soy milk
- Soy sauce
- Soy protein
- Tofu

Fermented soy products like tempeh, pickled tofu, natto, and soy miso are okay, as long as they are non-GMO.

Soy manufacturers have run such a successful marketing campaign that 75% of US consumers rate soy products as healthy.[12]

Gut health issues

If you want to preserve or foster your gut health, consider this:
- Soybeans can impair digestion of proteins because they contain enzyme inhibitors – enzymes are needed for protein digestion.[13]
- Consumption of soy products can lead to gastric distress[14] and soy has been shown to irritate the gut.
- As much as 90% of soy produced in the US today is genetically modified (GMO) and as a result contains the highest possible pesticide levels, usually glyphosate, which are toxic to the gut.

Other possible health issues of soy:
- Soy is a potent source of phytoestrogens which mimic estrogen and can lead to infertility and may promote breast cancer in adult women.

- Drinking two glasses of soy milk daily for as little as one month can alter a woman's menstrual cycle.
- Soy is high in goitrogens, substances which can block the normal functioning of the thyroid gland.
- The processing of soy produces cancer-causing nitrosamines.
- Soy foods contain high levels of aluminum, which is toxic to the nervous system.

Note: Infants must not be given soy milk (infant formula) as this can harm the sexual and reproductive development of the infant.

Weight loss claims

Soy proponents claim that some studies show that people who regularly consume soy protein tend to weigh less and have less abdominal fat than those who don't. They claim that soy isoflavones (estrogen-like substances) reduce belly fat and also protect against breast cancer.

This is nonsense!

Estrogenic compounds tend to increase belly fat and the presence of these isoflavones is one of the main reasons NOT to eat soy. As far as the breast cancer claim goes, a number of studies show that genistein (the main isoflavone) promotes the growth of breast cancer cells and tumors.

More reading

If you want to know more about the dangers of soy, I suggest you read *The Whole Soy Story* by Kaayla T. Daniel.

Good nuts and bad nuts

Nuts make good snacks when you feel you have to have something to eat. But there are good nuts and bad nuts. Bad nuts must be avoided and good nuts should be eaten in moderation.

Nuts allowed in moderation
- Macadamia (highest fat)
- Pecans
- Brazils
- Hazels
- Almonds

Nuts not allowed
- Peanuts
- Cashews
- Pistachios

As a matter of interest, cashews and pistachios also come from a bad family! They are cousins of the poison ivy (*anacardiaceae*) family.

Nuts and constipation

Yes, you can eat the good nuts above; just don't eat too many.

Nuts contain phytates in the form of phytic acid, which can cause constipation. If you are eating nuts and encounter some constipation, try stopping the nuts for a week and see if the constipation improves.

Phytates have a mixed bag of effects; they are good in the large intestine but not so good in the small intestine. I eat limited quantities of nuts often and if you can tolerate them, I think you should do so too.

Go easy on these!

Some foods have been proven to negatively influence psoriasis. A list of them is included on the following page.

Chilies

Besides being a nightshade, the alkaloids in chilies can increase the leakiness of your gut.[15] Avoid any bottled or commercial chili sauces because you have no idea what is in them. Bottled sauces also contain other ingredients that have no place in a healthy gut– things like preservative and gluten-containing flavorings.

During Detox, please do not eat any chilies either as a sauce or raw. Even on Maintenance I would go easy on these.

Peppers

Cayenne pepper is also bad in large quantities because of the capsaicin it contains.

Painkillers and anti-inflammatories

Before you reach for some pain relief, make sure that you need it. Obviously, sometimes pain relief is necessary, but be sure that you can't do without before swallowing the pills. Virtually all of these kinds of medication do some gut wall damage, so be careful to always use as little as possible.

When you do use painkillers, make sure you help the gut heal by drinking a few extra glasses of water with a teaspoon of L-Glutamine. Make yourself some slippery elm tea before bedtime; it is a powerful gut healer.

Instant coffee

Instant coffee contains chemicals and sometimes even gluten. Don't drink six to eight cups a day as so many people seem to do. Limit instant coffee use as much as you can and drink good quality filtered coffee instead.

Daily-use items to avoid

Here's a quick heads-up of products we often use without thinking, but should not.

- Skin care products
- Makeup and cosmetics
- Anti-bacterial soaps
- Commercial table salt
- Toothpaste and mouthwash
- Tinned foods
- Plastic bottles and containers
- Antacids
- Painkillers
- Overcooked foods

Note about EDTA: This is a preservative that often pops up in makeup and skin care products. Check the labels of the products you use regularly to see if they list EDTA. If they do, throw them out and find alternative products. EDTA acts as a 'penetration enhancer' on skin and gut surfaces. It makes them more leaky, which is precisely what we are trying to avoid.

Replace any skin care products that you can with glycerin containing versions. Glycerin (glycerol) is hugely beneficial for your skin.

Makeup and cosmetics

Be aware that certain makeup and cosmetic products contain ingredients that can be bad for your skin and your health. Cosmetics are often contaminated with heavy metals as demonstrated by a study that tested eye shadows. It showed that all of them contained traces of the heavy metals lead, cobalt, nickel, chromium, and arsenic.[16] Over 75% contained a higher amount of one of more of these metals.

Lipstick has even higher heavy metal levels, so use only when necessary. Many cosmetics have not even been tested.

If you wear makeup, I'm not saying that you stop completely. Instead, I suggest that you be parsimonious (cool word for thrifty) with your use of cosmetics. Who says you have to have makeup on all the time? Be natural whenever you can. The people who really love you will still love you!

Skin care products

Many of the dangers mentioned for makeup and cosmetics apply to skin care products such as:
- Soaps
- Deodorants
- Sunscreen
- Skin creams and moisturizers

Some of the suspect chemicals that you should be on the lookout for include:
- Triclosan
- Parabens (increase skin leakyness)
- Propylene glycol (irritates skin)
- Sodium lauryl sulfate (penetrates and irritates)

Be wary of any product that you use regularly; your skin care product may be contributing to your psoriasis. Watch for skin reddening or itching after use.

Anti-bacterial soaps and washes

We use these daily and most consumers will choose an 'anti-bacterial' version of a cleaning product ahead of a plain old version. Unfortunately most anti-bacterial soaps, cleaners and washes contain chemicals that you and the environment can do without.

Commercial table salt

Normal table salt comes with some additives that make it not completely natural. Remember that natural salt is not white! Most salt

of this kind has an anti-caking agent added to prevent the salt from clumping. These anti-caking agents can be:
- Calcium silicate
- Sodium alum inosilicate (contains aluminum)
- Magnesium carbonate (not regarded as toxic to eat, but burns the skin and eyes and causes gastric irritation if swallowed)

In addition, when a salt is iodized it usually has a potassium salt such as potassium iodide or sodium iodide added to it, along with some dextrose to prevent the potassium iodide from oxidizing.

There is too much legislative laxity around anti-caking agents for anyone trying to heal their gut to take a chance with them. Therefore, I recommend that you make use of pure sea salt or Himalayan salt crystals. The extra cost is well worth it.

Toothpaste

Normal off-the-shelf toothpaste is not the most wonderful stuff to put in your mouth or gut. It contains a number of chemicals that can worsen your psoriasis by damaging your gut. It should be obvious: never swallow toothpaste; in fact, washing your mouth out with water after brushing is probably a good idea. Consider switching to a natural toothpaste.

Here are some of the chemicals that may be in your toothpaste:

- Sodium fluoride, a poison that damages your gut and can cause nausea, vomiting or diarrhea. A Harvard University study found that it lowers children's IQ.[17] This is not the kind of stuff any sensible person would want near their body. This does not seem to worry the U.S. authorities. In 2012 so much fluoride was added to the U.S. water supply that a staggering 67% of people in America drank water with added sodium fluoride or fluorosilicic acid.[18]

- Dyes for coloring, which are often made from petroleum products.
- Foaming agents that make bubbles as you brush can be really deadly. The most common chemical for making bubbles is SLS (sodium laurel sulfate) and its derivatives. These potent chemicals have been linked to a number of reports that indicate increased cancer risks.
- Triclosan, a pesticide and antibacterial agent that has been linked to many health and environmental safety issues.
- Silica, an abrasive used to clean tooth enamel. It is also combined with cellulose in 'tooth whitening' products.

Mouthwash

Most commercial mouthwashes contain similar chemicals to the list above. Use it with caution and never swallow it.

Safety rules brushing teeth or using mouthwash

- Consider using an organic or natural product.
- Use a little as possible to get the job done.
- Never swallow the stuff.
- Spit it out properly, then rinse your mouth out with plenty of water and then spit that out too.

Tinned foods

Food sold in tins has no place in the diet of anyone who has an autoimmune disease. Food in tins is devoid of any live components. The tins are also lined with a protective plastic that further increases health risks. The plastic protective lining used in most food tins contains Bisphenol A (BPA) as well as other plastic pollutants. BPA has become a major health problem because it mimics natural hormones such as estrogen and disrupts hormone balance.

Plastic bottles and containers

These are bad for you! There is a huge commercial enterprise aimed at making and selling all manner of plastic utensils that are so convenient for us.

Plastic water bottles are a good example. You can use them over and over again, no problem. No! Plastic is made from chemicals that are really not good for you, one of which is BPA (as mentioned above). Don't pack or leave food in plastic wrap, unless you want the chemicals in the wrap to be part of your next meal.

Don't:
- Heat food in plastic containers as it greatly increases the levels of plasticizers in the food[19]
- Put warm food into a plastic container
- Use and especially re-use cheap plastic items. As a rule, the cheaper or flimsier the plastic the more dangerous it is to your health.

Whenever possible, store your food in glass containers.

Antacids

Many of these over-the-counter, so-called heartburn remedies contain aluminum, which can cause constipation.

Overcooked foods

Avoid cooking food at high temperatures, especially if cooked with vegetable oil (such as peanut, corn, and soy oil). Overheating food like eggs oxidizes cholesterol and turns it rancid.

DIET: MAINTENANCE

If you've gotten this far, well done! You have made it through the hard part of weaning yourself off grains and sugars and now need to settle into a routine and lifestyle that will keep you healthy for the rest of your life.

If you feel that you are missing out on a food treat or a specific dish that you loved, this phase allows you to slowly reintroduce some of the foods that you have been avoiding in Detox. But be careful, this phase can be dangerous.

If you don't feel that you're missing out, do your health a favor and just keep on doing all the stuff that you got used to in Detox.

Dangerous times

Make no mistake, the initial few months of Maintenance are the most dangerous time for you. You have achieved so much and it can all go down the drain very quickly.

Do you really want to look back at your achievements a year from now only to find that your skin lesions have slowly grown red and angry again?

Re-introducing some foods

Maintenance begins once your skin has healed sufficiently to your liking and your joints are feeling better. At this point, you can slowly re-introduce some of your favorite foods. There is a right way and a wrong way to do this.

The right way is to introduce one new food at a time. Monitor the effects of that new food for a week or two in order to ensure that you experience no ill effects.

What to watch for

- Watch carefully for joint pain and joint stiffness
- Check for new lesions that may pop up
- Ensure that any existing plaques do not get redder and are not raised or angry
- If at any time you get a sudden peeling or shedding of scabs, you must be cautious. Normally shedding like this means a change in the state of the disease. When this happens after you have added a new food to your diet, stop and remove it for a few weeks. Once your skin has settled down, you can try adding the suspicious food again but be extra alert.

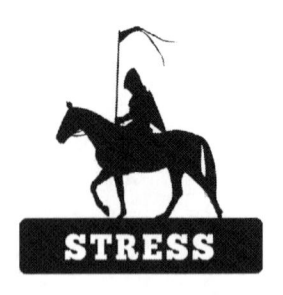

STRESS: The Second Horseman

The effects of stress

Please don't skip over this section just because you feel that there is nothing you can do to reduce your daily load of stress. There is.

You need to do some daily de-stressing to heal your psoriasis and to conserve your health. Learn from this section and you will be able to properly:
- Chill
- Chill out
- Relax
- Mellow out
- Unwind
- Loosen up

Sure, you know all the words, but do you know how to put them into action? To tame the Stress Horseman, you have to learn HOW to de-stress. I am going to show you some ways to do it as well as some tools that you can use daily.

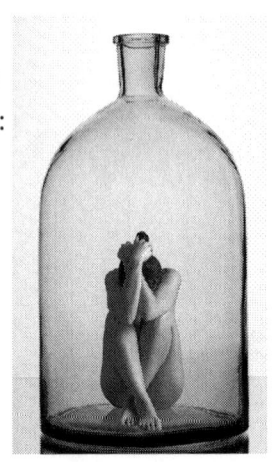

Use these tools regularly and you will tame the Second Horseman and at the same time:
- Age a lot slower
- Reduce your blood pressure
- Think more clearly
- Maybe even lose some weight

Since we all have different stressors and handle them in different ways, this section presents methods you can choose and adapt to work for you.

More stress makes more psoriasis

Everyone agrees that stress makes psoriasis worse. In some cases, it can trigger the disease. What's worse is that it works both ways, as anyone with the disease knows: having psoriasis causes stress! The more perceived stress you are under, the worse your psoriasis will be. The key to success is learning ways that you can use to help you manage your stress.

Chronic stress

My sister (bless her) uses the word chronic to mean 'bad'. To her chronic stress is a lot of stress. However, this is incorrect. In medical terms chronic simply means 'ongoing, never getting better'. Chronic stress is woven into the background noise of our daily lives.

Chronic stress is a threat to your health, the kind of threat that your body has no natural tools to deal with. Instead, you are wired to react to sudden life or death events, the kinds of challenges that are resolved in seconds or minutes. For example, a lion chases you causing you stress and as a consequence to run or hide. Whatever you do, your stress levels will drop soon after.

The opposite occurs in modern life. Most of our stressors are ever-present such as traffic, lines, financial worries, family pressures and the rest. These chronic stresses cause our engines to be fueled by something they were never designed to run on.

Cortisol, the stress hormone

Cortisol is the fuel of stress. Despite being involved in many functions in the body, such as maintaining blood pressure levels and regulation of the immune system, cortisol and adrenaline are also key players in the body's reaction to stress. As a result cortisol is known as the 'stress hormone'. Chronic stress can be measured in the blood and shows up as high cortisol and low DHEA levels.

When cortisol is squirted into the blood during an immediately stressful situation, it acts to slow digestion and reduce gut absorption. Blood is diverted from the gut to the muscles, where it can do more immediate good. This action seems sensible when the aim is to stay alive and the gut can digest the food later. However, when cortisol levels in the blood remain chronically high, the gut becomes leaky, which worsens your psoriasis.

You can get your doctor to measure your cortisol levels, often done with a simple spit test. Blood cortisol levels usually mirror stress levels, which can be monitored periodically to measure how well your stress management is working.

The effects of stress

Chronic or unremitting stress has many negative long-term effects on your body. These include:
- A weakened immune system
- Faster aging
- Leaky gut

- Reduced ability of the gut to absorb nutrients and minerals and the knock-on effects of these deficiencies.

Stress affects your entire body

Many internal body processes are 'automatic' and proceed without our knowledge or control. The nervous system controlling these functions is called the Autonomic Nervous System (ANS). Examples of organs under ANS control include the heart, gut, lungs and pupils of the eye.

The ANS has two parts: one part that slows things down and another that speeds things up. Under ideal conditions, both systems are in equilibrium but in stressful conditions control shifts to the 'speed me up' (fight or flight) system. This results in the typical 'stressed out' state we so often exist in. These two systems are called the sympathetic and parasympathetic nervous systems.

Some indicators of a stressed state include:
- Clenched jaw
- Racing thoughts and a sense of urgency
- Rapid shallow breathing
- Neck and shoulder muscle stiffness
- Angry or tearful outbursts

The stress reduction strategies outlined in this section strive to reduce the influence of your unconscious 'fight or fight' dominance in favor of the more restful 'feed and breed' system.

Stress affects your gut

Stress can affect your gut. Think of that queasy feeling you had before the big exam or the loss of appetite and maybe even explosive diarrhea before the big interview. Some of us lose our appetite in stressful situations; others can't stop eating. Either way, it's the gut telling the brain how to act.

Simply thinking of a stressful incident or replaying a social slight can affect your body. As the negative thought goes through your mind, your blood pressure rises, blood is diverted away from your gut and digestion slows down.

A recent study looked at how common stress, like multitasking, affects the gut. The test subjects spoke on the phone and at the same time tried to listen to someone standing next to them asking them a question. This is a situation we all can relate to. The researchers then measured the change in mineral absorption in each test subject's gut. What they found was astounding. The stress of trying to multitask halved the gut absorption in the test subjects.

What's more, the absorption deficit persisted for over two hours, even after the stress was withdrawn. It does not take much imagination to apply this one simple stress and its effects to what happens to your gut on a typical Monday morning.

Surprisingly, stress also affects the bugs living in our gut.[20] They feel our stress and a stressful event can decimate gut bacterial populations, similar to what happens on a larger scale to soldiers in combat. A Russian study of pilots in dangerous combat missions found that the stress of combat could totally wipe out all the bugs in a pilot's gut.

Adrenal stress

Cortisol, the stress hormone, is produced by your adrenal glands. Normally your adrenals will raise cortisol levels during a sudden emergency. This response is aimed at boosting your energy levels so that you can escape the emergency. However, the stress of modern life causes an overproduction of cortisol and some people live their lives with elevated levels of cortisol, which is really bad for their health.

It is said that 'the adrenals listen to what your heart tell your brain'. This means that lower, steadier heart rates drop your cortisol levels and thus lowers your stress. Many of the stress management methods I suggest also do exactly that.

Stress makes you old

Stress does more than harm your psoriasis; it makes you age faster. It has been shown that there is a strong relationship between perceived stress and the rate at which you age.[21] Elizabeth Blackburn measured stress at a cellular level, using mothers caring for their children in ICU. Her data indicated that they aged about ten years faster than women who did not have to deal with this kind of stress.

Stress also:
- Harms your heart.
- Makes you fat.
- Weakens your immune system.
- Damages your brain and nervous system.

Managing your relationship with stress

Fact: You cannot avoid stress. So often we hear well-meaning stress management advice that cautions us 'to avoid stress'. Unfortunately, this is impossible for most of us to do. Stress is part of modern life and can only be avoided by impractical means, such as retreating to a cave in the wilderness.

Root out the little stresses of daily life

The first step you can take is to identify things that stress you in daily life and where possible make adjustments to reduce them. As a first step write down your stressors; identify the ones that you have control over and fix them as best you can.

For example, if you find the traffic on the way to work stressful, make an arrangement to avoid it. If missing deadlines is stressful, find a way to do your work on time. Just the act of recognizing the small things that stress you is a step in the right direction.

Ways to de-stress

Here are some great ways to de-stress. Try them out and see which ones work best for you. My list is not exhaustive; please add your own methods if you need to. I have, however, specified some non-negotiable de-stress techniques, which I call the Must Dos. You have to try to make these a part of your lifestyle in the future.

There is also a section of other suggested options that you can choose from. If you have any favorites that I have not mentioned, please mail them to me at 4horsemen@biohacks.guru.

Must do

- Control your breathing
- Eat mindfully
- Control your self-talk

Strongly suggested

- Get back to nature
- Nurture your friendships and relationships
- Get hugged every day
- Meditate
- Go on a Low-Info diet
- Eat dark chocolate
- Sweat

Breathing control

Slow or controlled breathing is an effective way to reduce stress. Regular slow breaths signal your brain that all is well and if done properly, will induce a relaxation response. In this way, you can convert the rapid, shallow breathing of someone under stress to that of a relaxed person.

Controlled breathing is often the result of many stress-relieving activities like meditation, prayer, reading a book, listening to music. Once you learn a controlled breathing technique, you can use it when you stress out to tell your brain that you are OK. You can use it as often as you like – it will work for you in the traffic, in bed or in the office.

The relaxation response

This term, coined by Dr Herbet Benson in the 1970s, was based on his work, which suggested that we have a natural response designed to relax us, just as we have the fight or flight response.[22] He believed that a mental device such as a sound, a prayer, staring at a scene and adopting a passive attitude that put stressful thoughts aside, would produce relaxation, irrespective of the circumstances. This meant that it could be used anywhere, not just in quiet situations. Today even mainstream medicine agrees with him and has found similar benefits. An example is Breath Focus, presented in a 2015 article published by the Harvard Medical School, which describes a breath control method to lower stress levels.[23]

Control your breath to:
- Reduce stress
- Lower anxiety levels
- Drop blood pressure
- Lower heart rate

Making time for breath control

Breath control is a vital tool in your stress management toolbox. Have you ever seen Captain America in action? He uses his brightly painted shield to deflect sharp objects intended to harm him. Breath control is your shield.

Use your stress shield as you feel your stress begin to rise. Do it too at other times convenient for you, such as in your car in the traffic, before you start work or a meeting, and in bed. Another really important time is just before meals; it only takes a few seconds and will improve digestion and enjoyment of the meal.

Signs that you are winning

Controlled breathing stimulates the 'rest and relax' part of your nervous system. When you do it properly, you may feel some physical sensations such as a running nose, rosy face or a sense of body warmth. If you often feel cold, breathing like this will help to warm you up.

Buteyko breathing

I want to teach you a 'lite' version of Buteyko breathing. Ukrainian physiologist, Konstantin Buteyko, developed it as an asthma treatment, but it also has great value in other areas.

Buteyko believed that the modern lifestyle and open-mouth breathing leads to higher carbon dioxide levels in the blood. Higher carbon dioxide levels constrict blood vessels and reduce oxygen levels in places like the hands and feet. When you breathe the Buteyko way, you warm up, think clearer and have higher energy levels and better sleep patterns.

Nose breathing is the key, because it lowers carbon dioxide levels and raises nitrous oxide levels, which opens the lung passages and improves blood flow. It will almost always unblock blocked noses.

You are in no danger of running out of oxygen

Buteyko breathing will not affect your oxygen levels!

Your urge to breathe is driven by levels of carbon dioxide in your blood. If these are too high, they will unnecessarily reduce the pauses between your breaths, making you over-breathe. Over time, breathing the Buteyko way will give you better body oxygenation and lower stress levels.

Test your carbon dioxide levels

Here is a simple way for you to find out if your carbon dioxide levels are too high. It can be done anywhere and at almost any time. All you need is a timer with a second hand.

Here's how to do it:
- Sit comfortably on a chair
- Breathe out normally
- Use thumb and finger to pinch your nose closed
- Start timing
- Hold your breath
- Wait until you feel the first definite desire to take a breath
- Read the timer
- Let go of your nose and breathe in

It is not a 'hold your breath' contest! What you are measuring is the time it takes before you consciously feel the need to take a breath. If you were in a breath holding competition, you could hold your breath for much longer.

A control pause of 20 seconds or less points to a high carbon dioxide level, over 25 is fair and over 30 seconds is a good result.

It is not a sign of fitness. In fact, most fit people have poor control pauses because they over-breathe when they train. I tested some elite cyclists last year and once they stopped trying to win the breath-holding contest, most of them came in at 15 seconds or below. As fit as they were, their breathing was driven by carbon dioxide and once they trained using Buteyko methods, most of them had improved race performances.

Work on your control pause

I work on my control pause all day! So should you.

Do this often: Whenever you have a moment during the day, consciously don't breathe in and when you feel the urge to take a breath, wait an extra few seconds before you do. Over time the gap between your breaths will increase and so will your control pause.

Buteyko breathe all the time

Here's how to do controlled breathing the Buteyko way.

First, I suggest that you breathe through your nose all the time or at least as often as you can manage. Second, do the exercise below when you need to de-stress or are about to eat a meal, go to bed, and so on.

Points to remember:
- You can do this anywhere
- Always breathe through your nose
- Never take full chest stretching breaths in
- Never force all the air out of your lungs
- You don't have to hold your nose if you don't want to

Buteyko controlled breathing exercise

- Get as comfortable as you can
- Close your mouth

- Take a normal, relaxed breath in and out through your nose (don't breathe deeply)
- Now hold your breath or block your nose and do a slow mental count down from five to one
- Then unblock your nose and take a gentle breath in and out
- Hold your breath again or block your nose for a slow count of five (NB: If you find this pause difficult, you can reduce or omit the pause; it is important to breathe comfortably)
- Repeat this process for between two to four minutes
- If you become short of breath, keep breathing gently until you feel comfortable again

There are many online resources that will provide you with more detail about this method.

Nadi Shodhana (Nadi Shodan)

Nadi shodhana is from pranayama, Sanskrit for the 'extension of life energy through breath'. We will learn a version of pranayama that uses the nose (nadi) purification (shodhana). It has a similar action to the Buteyko method discussed above.

Also known as Alternate Nostril Breathing, nadi shodhana is a form of breathing that has been shown to produce relaxation and reduce heart rate. It has also been found to have beneficial effects on heart rate variability[24] as well as on improving problem-solving abilities.

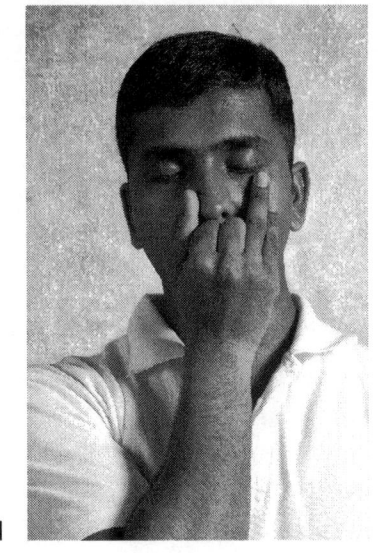

In this method you rhythmically alternate breathing between the left and right nostrils, with pauses between both in and out breaths. There are many YouTube videos showing the technique; browse through them and find a method that you're comfortable with.

Mindful eating

Don't eat on the move!

Never grab a quick bite, and don't eat when you're stressed. Rushed eating sends a message to your gut telling it that you are under stress. Whatever you do, don't do it like this guy!

A brilliant example

During a video lecture, Marc David, a specialist in the psychology of eating, recounts the story of one of his patients, Dr X.[25] Dr X believed that he ate well but nevertheless experienced intense indigestion after every meal. Despite having access to many medical specialists, he had lived with abdominal discomfort for almost twenty years. Dr X's daily fare was McDonald's for breakfast and lunch, eaten in his car in the McDonald's parking lot, in order to save time. For dinner, he would consume a take-out, sitting in front of the TV.

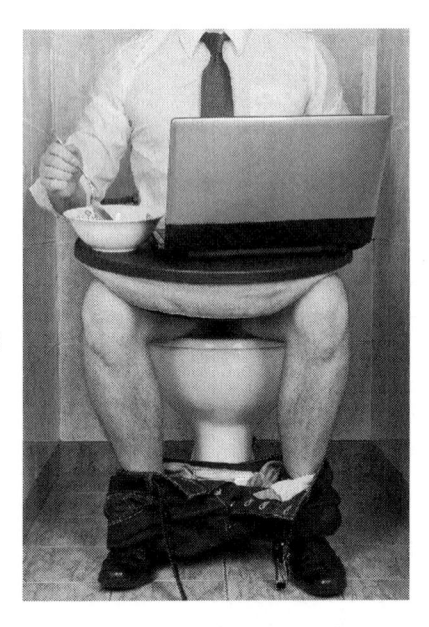

He insisted that he was happy with his lifestyle and would not consider changing it. Amazingly, Marc David did not try to persuade the patient to eat healthy food (as I would have). What he prescribed was a simple eating slow-down. All he asked the patient to do was to take longer with each of his junk food meals and to slow down with some deep breaths before starting to eat.

Two weeks later Dr X called Marc to say that his digestive issues were completely cured. On top of this, once he had slowed his eating down, he found that he could actually taste the Big Macs, which now tasted terrible to him, and he switched to healthier food as a result.

Slow down when you eat

Eating under duress – be it anxiety, time pressures or any other stressor – is bad for your gut. Tests done to study stressful eating have shown that it can reduce absorption by as much as 50%, for up to two hours afterward.

You are stress eating, when you eat:
- On the run
- Standing up
- In the car
- Quickly
- On autopilot

Eating mindfully

The concept of mindful eating comes from Buddhist teachings about how to eat. Before eating, Buddhists consider the food they are about to eat and where it comes from. They also chew their food carefully, savoring the tastes and textures.

Marc David suggests a pause to regulate breathing before starting to eat. You could use the Buteyko technique mentioned in the Breathing Control section, or just simply, mindfully slow your breathing. Try to be present in the act of eating. Don't eat on autopilot, not even tasting the food you swallow.

How to eat mindfully

- Control your breathing
- Consider the food on your plate; try to be grateful for what is in front of you
- Be present in your act of eating
- Chew each mouthful properly
- Feel the texture of your food; explore the taste of it
- Make a conscious effort to slow down

Control your self-talk

> **'Don't let the noise of others' opinions drown out your own inner voice.'**
>
> *Steve Jobs*

Ever done any self-attacking?

You know, those times when you think mean thoughts about yourself or insult and undermine yourself. I suppose we are all guilty of doing this from time to time but if it's the norm, then this kind of behavior is bad for your stress levels and at the same time bad for your psoriasis.

Self-attacking ties in with self-esteem. Self-esteem is about how you see yourself, your skills, abilities and overall value. Your level of self-esteem not only guides your behavior, it has also been shown to predict health and wellbeing.[26]

If you have a poor opinion of yourself or if you have a tendency to berate and insult yourself, then you have to work on this area in order to manage and reduce your stress levels. Additionally, this kind of behavior reduces your ability to handle other stressful situations that you may have to deal with as part of daily life.

Frame your self-attacker as someone else

Next time you have a self-attacking thought, stop and ask yourself; what if someone else had said that to you? Would you think differently about it then?

Then think about this: How would you feel if you had someone following you around all day berating you with negative personal comments? Would you tolerate having this sort of person around you? Surely you would soon grow tired of the haranguing and negativity and try your best to avoid their bad company?

There is no reason to tolerate this type of behavior, especially if you are inflicting it on yourself!

Restricting self-criticism

- Do you think that you are hard on yourself?
- Do you tend to color events and issues in a negative light?

Read these words:
- Useless
- Pathetic

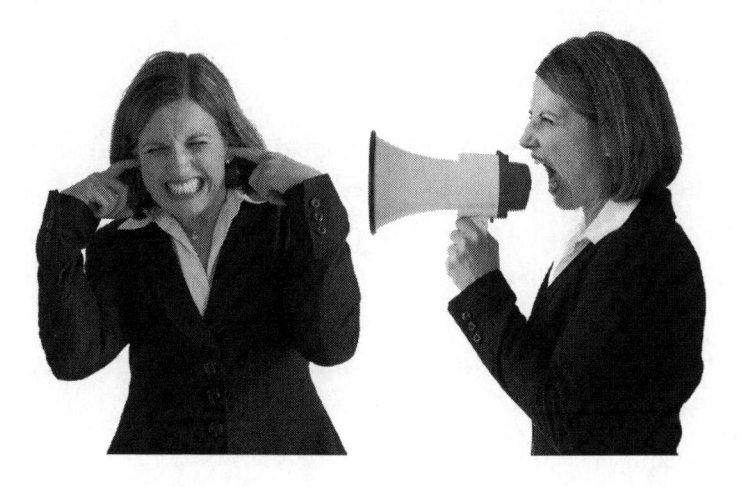

- Stupid
- Worthless
- Ugly
- Inadequate

Does thinking about any of these words make you feel bad?[27]

Well, you shouldn't feel that way. Self-criticism is not a good thing. Trust yourself and always choose praise over criticism. I ask the question again: 'Are you too hard on yourself?'

> *'Too many people undervalue what they are, and overvalue what they're not.'*
> INTERNET POSTCARD

Dr Melanie Fennell is a recognized expert on low self-esteem and she suggests that the best way to handle self-critical thoughts is with a three-step process:

Recognize, question, re-frame

1. Recognize each negative thought

Catch the thoughts as they happen. Although you may find recognition to be difficult at first, be alert, because self-critical thoughts can be triggered by certain situations or mental images. Learn to take notice of when you start feeling down about yourself. If you find this difficult, Fennel suggests setting an alarm to go off at one-hour intervals and using this as the cue to ask yourself if you have had any self-critical thoughts over the past 60 minutes.

2. Question each negative thought

Ask yourself 'why' using questions and try to seek a balanced alternative. You can try to do this as a trial lawyer questioning a witness would by asking yourself:
- Are you certain of your facts?
- Are you jumping to conclusions?
- Are you being too hard on yourself and too easy on others?
- Are you taking the blame for things that were not your fault?
- Are you thinking in black and white, and allowing yourself no leeway?

3. Re-frame each negative thought

Review your negative thoughts in a positive way. Then act according to the new way that you are looking at them. Always treat yourself with respect.

Example: 'I'm useless, I only came fifth overall.'
Re-framed: 'Nice job! I came in fifth and I just started playing.'

Of course, it is important not to lose touch with reality, but putting a positive spin on things helps. Yes, you need to face your failures but cast them as learning experiences and as some bad luck that has been personally directed at you.

Recognize biased thinking

We naturally add weight to ideas and thoughts that are consistent with our beliefs, just as we diminish those that aren't. Don't you hate people who openly show bias or prejudice? People who start sentences with: 'I can't stand ...'

Now what if you are biased against yourself? What if by default you perceive thoughts about yourself as well as events that happen to you in a negative way? Why do such a bad thing to yourself? Recognizing and removing this inbuilt bias will make a huge difference to your self-esteem.

Don't think in a self-limiting way

'I can't do that!' How often have you told yourself that?

Love the skin you're in

You've heard it before: 'If you don't love yourself, then who will?' There is no way to get a body transplant and the only way you are ever going to leave your body is when you die. So you need to accept, love and appreciate yourself.

Give yourself credit

If you do well at something, take a mental bow. Give yourself the credit. Don't be so quick to give the credit to luck, to someone else, or even to the intervention of a deity. Give yourself a pat on the back.

Avoid the perfect

Nothing in life is perfect. Neither are you, so cut yourself some slack and don't always expect yourself to be perfect. Everybody has blemishes and bad days and you're allowed to have them too. Don't ever allow yourself to recognize criticism as failure.

Be confident

Did you know that you can train yourself to have more self-confidence? If you think that you lack confidence, consider taking a self-confidence course. There are many available online and some of them are even free.

Here are some pointers to consider:
- Remember your achievements and successes; make a list and read it if you feel your confidence slipping.
- Make a list of your personal goals and tick off any that you achieve.
- Divide your goals into small steps and focus on one step at a time.
- Celebrate each success as you tick it off.
- Get your support network involved in your successes and failures.
- Smile at yourself in the mirror.

Back to nature

> '... being connected to nature and feeling happy are, in fact, connected.'
>
> *From a study of nature connectedness and happiness*[28]

When last were you outdoors?

Our roots as humans are deeply embedded in the outdoors. However, most of us spend almost no time outside, even though contact with nature makes us happy in such an elemental way. Contact with nature is not optional. We need this kind of connectedness, which we can never reproduce by immersing ourselves in a life of materialism or machines.

What is nature?

Nature is more than the plants and trees we find outdoors. Animals and weather are also an important part of nature. As humans, we are hardwired to connect with other mammals. Think of your emotions when seeing baby animals, how you feel when looking into the eyes of a puppy or lion cub.

Nature is also weather. We control our living environments so tightly that it abstracts us from the real weather outdoors. Granted, the weather outdoors may be sometimes unpleasant; hot, humid, cold or wet. How do you feel when you think of a sunny day, a gloomy sky or walking in the rain? Maybe we need to experience the feeling of being too hot or too cold?

Exposure to nature

Spending time in natural surroundings restores some of our capacity to handle the emotional and psychological stresses in our daily lives.

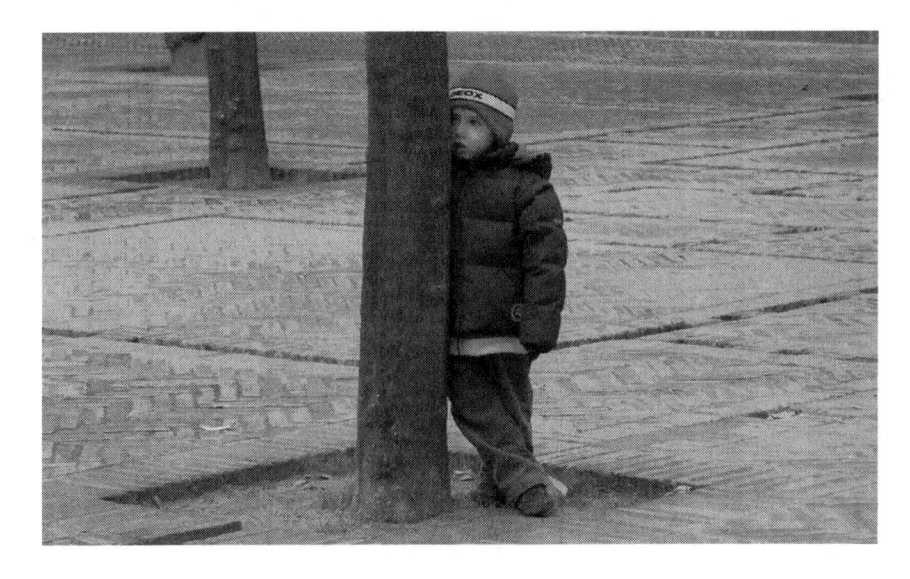

It works this way for adults and kids alike. A Swedish study found that children who spent time playing outdoors closer to nature showed better development in the areas of learning and understanding (cognitive development) than kids who played in concrete jungles.[29]

The ability to control our moods and to delay gratification is called self-regulation. Francis Ming Kuo, professor of Natural Resources and Environmental Sciences, says that our ability to self-regulate is enhanced by being outdoors. She says this is an essential component of good health.[30]

Practical steps to de-stress outdoors

I hope that by having read the two paragraphs above, you fully appreciate how much your health and your psoriasis needs you to spend some time outdoors! When you do get the chance to be outdoors, do it barefoot – this will magnify your connection.

My wife

My wife recently started on a mindfulness, back-to-nature journey that I initially poo-pooed. We are lucky to live in the suburbs in a house that has a garden and a small outdoor living area; an area that we have in the past spent very little time living in. She changed all that. She started spending time in the garden during the day and also at night-time. I joined her, initially just to be polite, as I would normally work or watch TV indoors before bedtime. These days, I never wear shoes at home, whereas in the past the only time I would walk barefoot was on my way to bed. I put my cell phone away, seldom watch TV and rather spend my time outside. We often just lie on the grass and look at the stars, an activity I would have considered crazy in the past. It has worked for me; I can't believe how much more relaxed I feel and how much more I am enjoying life at home.

Depending on your situation, getting to a park or a natural outdoor environment may not be so simple. If you live in a concrete environment, where the only green stuff around you is the vegetable aisle in the supermarket, then you need to be creative in finding ways to chill out in nature. Is there a park or a rooftop garden you can retreat to? Make a plan. There has to be a way for you to get your bare feet in the grass or your skin in the sun a few times a week.

Find a safe place where you can either sit outdoors, lie on the ground and read a book, or stare into space. You don't always need company to do this; sometimes the solitude of being alone is a tonic.

Don't stress too much about the weather. If it's cold outside, dress warmly but still do it! If it's too hot, just relax and sweat a little – it's good for you.

Walk barefoot

> **'The research done to date supports the concept that grounding or earthing the human body may be an essential element in the health equation along with sunshine, clean air and water, nutritious food, and physical activity.'**
>
> *Journal of Environmental and Public Health*[31]

Read that quote carefully. It was written by a group of scientific specialists whose skills include cell biology, cardiology and neurosurgery.

Our modern footwear insulates us from the earth. The Grounding Movement maintain that being in contact with the earth is a critical part of wellness. They maintain that grounding (or earthing) by walking barefoot allows for the transfer of electrons from the earth's surface into our bodies, balancing us electrically.[32] Ever since humans walked the planet, this was our natural state.

Obviously, this is not something that most mainstream medical practitioners accept, but since walking barefoot in nature is one of my prescriptions for stress management, what do you have to lose by trying it? Get out of your shoes whenever you get the chance.

Love your pet

If you don't have a pet, maybe you should consider getting one? Or if you do, then spend more time with your pet – it will do you both a power of good. Spending time with other people's pets also works.

Nurture friendships and relationships

I am sure that you already know that good friendships and family relationships are important. When your relationships go well, they can be a great de-stressor. When things go wrong in your relationships, they can also be a source of great stress.

The science is clear: Better relationships translate into lower stress levels. The problem is: How do we conduct and maintain better relationships? Like any other action in your de-stress mission, you are going to have to work at it. And like so many things in life, the more sustained the effort you make, the better will be the results.

Friendships take effort and time. They also require turning the other cheek occasionally. Family relationships are even harder but quality family time is always good for you and your stress levels.

> '**External relationships are improved and maintained through your expression of acceptance, peace, compassion and respect for all individuals in your environment...**'
>
> *From the book* Managing Stress[33]

Try to connect with others emotionally, spiritually and mentally. Don't isolate yourself at home or at work – the stress of this may lead to feelings of depression and isolation. Wherever possible, surround yourself with like-minded people who make you feel good.

Avoid negative energy in your life. You must know people who drain you and suck your positive energy? Avoid them. Don't be afraid to duck invitations to events you would rather not attend. Be like the parent in the aircraft safety drill: first put the oxygen mask on your own face before looking after other passengers around you.

Think carefully about the suggestions on the next page. They will help you build better relationships and a committed support system that will be there for you whenever you need to de-stress.

Try to:
- Be respectful to everyone around you
- Be kind to others
- Give credit to others
- Be positive toward your friends and family
- Forgive; let go of meaningless offenses and slights
- Learn to receive from others by being less fearful and more open and accepting
- Don't be afraid to ask for help

Get hugged daily

Hugging is good for you! It's a scientific fact that hugging is good medicine. A good hug releases oxytocin. Patting a dog does too. Oxytocin is a stress reduction hormone.[34] It works its magic by dropping blood cortisol levels.

Boost your oxytocin every day

This is one de-stressor that you should consciously work at boosting. Hugging is one way and there are a number of others, including:

- Holding hands
- Having an orgasm
- Getting a massage
- Giving a backrub
- Doing breathing exercises and meditation
- Getting touched lightly
- Giving or receiving praise

Dr Love's eight hugs a day

Paul Zak is probably the most enthusiastic oxytocin fan on the planet. He is also known as Dr Love because of his advice to always hug people as a means of raising oxytocin levels. If you want to know more about Dr Love, watch his TED talk 'Paul Zak: Trust, morality – and oxytocin'. It has been watched over a million times.

Dr Love suggests that to keep your oxytocin levels high and thus lower your stress, you should make sure that you are hugged eight times a day. I am not sure if you can achieve that but there is no harm in trying!

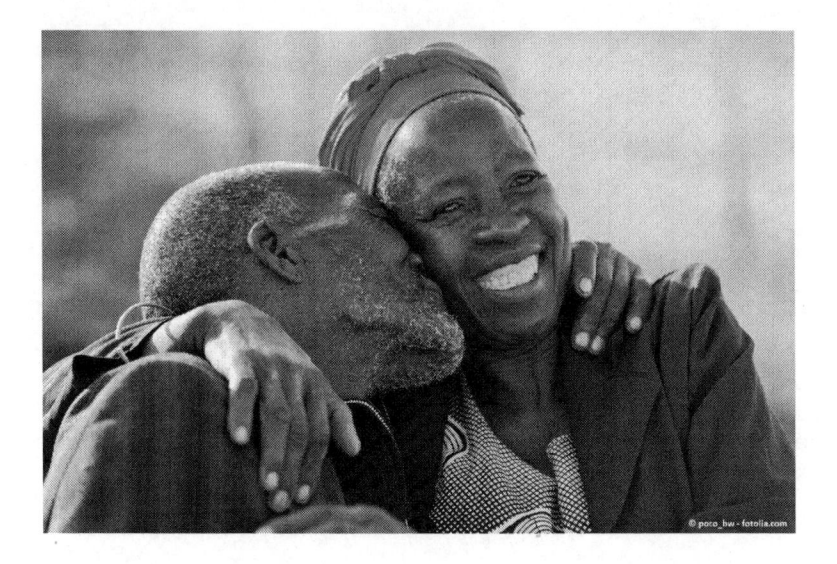

Meditate

For stressful daily situations use the breathing control methods explained in the section before this one. Meditation (for beginners at least) requires a quiet place as well as the intention to relax and quieten the mind.

If you don't meditate yet, now is the time to start! It will lower your stress levels and help your body deal with the psoriasis. Meditation has been shown by medical studies as well as by countless personal experiences to lower blood pressure, protect heart health, improve digestion (yes that's the gut we're trying to heal) and boost immunity.

There are literally thousands of ways to meditate and a myriad of schools that teach it. If you are new to meditation, there are many teaching resources you can use. You can also find a local teacher or a group to join. There are many courses and apps online that you can download.

You can also combine mediation with controlled breathing, discussed in the previous section.

The Six-Phase Meditation Method (Envisioning Method)

I am going to outline a simple six-step method developed by an entrepreneur and philanthropist, Vishen Lakhiani. He runs a website called Mindvalley Academy, which has many useful resources. One of these is his Six Phase Meditation Method, also called the Envisioning Method, which he says is a distillation of hundreds of books on personal growth. He calls it (rather modestly) 'The world's simplest, science-based, meditation and mindfulness technique'.

There is a full video explanation by Vishen on YouTube, which you can find by going to YouTube and searching for his name and "Six Phase Meditation Method" or "Envisioning Method".

Here in brief are the six steps.

Preparation: Relaxation
Lack of tension and comfort is your goal. Sit in a comfortable chair or lie flat on your back with your head on a small pillow. Play some calming instrumental music at a low volume.

Then physically relax your body. Start by relaxing your scalp and once it has relaxed, relax your eyelids, then flow gently down your body, relaxing each part as you go.

1. Connection
Focus on your consciousness; see it as a white light surrounding your body. Expand the light to encompass your suburb, then your town, then the world. Try to feel part of the whole.

2. Gratitude
Think of some of the things you should be grateful for, savor these things and feel the gratitude throughout your body.

3. Forgiveness
Think of someone who has done you wrong. Try to imagine them in front of you, apologize and ask for their forgiveness. Then forgive them.

4. Visualizing success
Think of how you would like your life to turn out over the next few years. Feel how much better things will become in your life.

5. Daily intention
Visualize your day ahead; consider the things that you will enjoy during the day. See today as a wonderful gift.

6. Blessing

Summon your inner strength or the strength of a higher power. Ask for support. Ask for luck and energy. Feel the support as your protective energy.

Now slowly bring yourself out of your meditation.

Go on a Low-Info diet

From the moment we wake until our eyes close at night we are bombarded with news. Does knowing this news help your life in any way? Does allowing yourself to be distracted by the whims of our sensationalist media serve you in any positive way?

Ask yourself this question: How much do you really need to know about foreign wars, terror attacks, lost planes, business indicators or the personal tragedies and triumphs of people you will never meet?

> '... we invented a toxic form of knowledge called 'news'. News is to the mind what sugar is to the body: appetizing, easy to digest – and highly destructive in the long run.'
>
> *Rolf Dobelli* – The Art of Thinking Clearly

I strongly suggest that you consider going on an information diet as a stress management practice. It worked for me.

My Low-Info diet

From the beginning of the year, I stopped listening to all news – cold turkey. For the past few years, I permanently had a screen open on my laptop, streaming news from a 24-hour Internet news station. I would constantly flip between my work and the news feed, as if I was eager to read about some world-shattering event before the people around me could. Of course, I also had a news app on my smart phone and my car radio was permanently jammed on a 24-hour news station to ensure that I would miss nothing as I was driving.

Well, I stopped doing this and now I no longer float between the news website and my work. When I drive, classical music wafts out of my car stereo and I make a conscious effort not to get angry in the traffic. I try to be courteous and, where possible, make eye contact with other drivers and pedestrians. At home, the TV in my bedroom is unplugged and I eschew the addictive call of the news channels.

This makes me thoroughly under-informed. I rely on the people around me to tell me of earth-shattering events and, most importantly, I don't waste time stressing about events that I have no control over.

The net effect of my information diet is that my stress levels are lower and I concentrate better on my work. I can now think almost as clearly as Rolf Dobelli.

Your Low-Info diet

Review your habits when it comes to the news and information. Think about how much time you spend reading news articles, blog posts and watching video news clips. Tune-out from these as much as you can. Stop reading the newspapers.

While you're at it, think about your social media habits. If you are anything like so many of my patients, you probably spend too much time trawling Facebook and similar websites. Some people I know slavishly watch Twitter feeds, waiting for the opportunity to tweet something pithy and profound.

I am not suggesting that you delete your Facebook account! Rather, apply a sensible compromise that will work for you. Limit the time you spend on social media. Don't blindly go down rabbit holes dug by people who have too much time on their hands. Realize that you will run out of life long before the denizens of Facebook will run out of pointless, funny videos for you watch.

Eat dark chocolate

Besides the benefits to your heart from eating dark chocolate, there is also some scientific evidence to show that dark chocolate is effective in lowering stress.

Dark chocolate need-to-know

Before you rush off to buy some, there are a few important things that you need to know.

Avoid any dark chocolate that has too much sugar in it. Many varieties of dark chocolate are similar to the popular brands in terms of high sugar milk chocolate. The dark chocolate you need to look for is normally clearly labeled with a cacao (cocoa) percentage. Go for the brands containing 80% or more of cacao. The higher the cacao percentage, the less sugar comes along for the ride and the more effective the chocolate will be at lowering stress.

My favorite dark chocolate is Lindt 85%, which has a high cocoa content and a meager 1g of sugar in each square.

Unfortunately, the low sugar levels give this kind of chocolate a bitter taste. For eaters of 'normal' chocolate, this takes a bit of getting used to. Instead of starting with the 85% variety, rather work your way towards it by first eating 65% or 70% cacao for a few weeks. Initially these may also be a little bitter, but stick to it for a few weeks before venturing into the higher percentages.

Stress busting

A few studies have reported cortisol-lowering effects in test subjects. The initial study was done by researchers at the Nestlé Research Center, which raised some eyebrows about impartiality.[35] However, a subsequent study done in 2014 showed similar results.[36] They reported that eating some dark chocolate before a stressful event has an effect on the adrenal glands and reduces the levels of cortisol (the stress hormone) produced during the event.

I think that we can safely assume that dark chocolate has some de-stressing effect, which it exerts by reducing cortisol levels. I suggest that you indulge in a few squares of dark chocolate a few times a week, preferably after dinner when you are winding down.

Sweat!

'Sauna bathers most frequently cite stress reduction as the number one benefit of sauna use.'

I thought long and hard about calling regular sauna sessions a 'must do' stress buster. It is that important. A regular sweat will be good for your stress levels and your psoriasis.

We try our hardest to avoid sweating. Is just not done to sweat in polite company. People use anti-perspirants to block sweat glands and meet in rooms with air conditioners. From Hollywood's perspective, sweating is usually a sign of guilt. They often show scenes where the perpetrator pours sweat, while the cops interrogating him are bone dry.

Sweat more when you can; it helps to excrete heavy metals from your body, which will improve your psoriasis. In the right environment, sweating also reduces stress. I strongly recommend that you consider using the sauna and steam room as part of your de-stress program. Use your time in the hot room to relax; it's a good time to use your meditation technique to further help relax your mind and body.

Some caution is required though; start slowly and increase your time in the hot room gradually. It is also prudent to have someone with you when you start in case you feel faint.

Important: After-sauna skin care

I have found that rubbing pure glycerin into hot skin after a steam or sauna session produces remarkable results. Apply immediately after showering, while your skin is still warm from the sauna. If you find the pure glycerin too sticky, you can dilute your glycerin by pre-mixing it with some water. The glycerin can reduce or clear skin plaques and seems to reduce wrinkles and rejuvenate normal skin. The only downside is that it leaves the skin slightly sticky, a small price to pay for the results it produces.

Worsens psoriasis?

I read a patient testimonial about a forty-year-old who found that a weekly sauna cleared his psoriasis. Others say that it makes their skin worse. If this happens to you, try to be persistent and keep going two or three times a week for a few consecutive weeks. The redness often goes away, but if you are still having a bad reaction after that, it is probably best to stop.

Bad press

When I grew up, it seemed that steam rooms were somewhat sleazy places where old men and creeps sat and whispered under the cover of steam. Saunas had a better reputation, but were less common. Even today, the saunas in the gyms I frequent are often empty during the day.

However, having spent quite some time visiting saunas and steam rooms over the past few years, I have made a complete reversal and now consider them to be some of the friendliest and most relaxing places to spend time in. The people I meet, sitting semi-naked and pouring sweat, are almost invariably friendly. I often ask them why they do it and most of them say that it's the best part of their day.

Tom Cruise and the sauna

After the 911 catastrophe, many of the firefighters and emergency personnel who worked at Ground Zero were found to have high blood levels of heavy metals like arsenic, cadmium, lead, and mercury. This was thought to be a result of their inhalation of toxin-laced smoke and dust from the burning materials in the buildings.

In 2003, Tom Cruise co-founded the New York Rescue Workers Detoxification Project, which gave these exposed workers access to a Scientology method for detoxification called the Purification Rundown. This has received both good and bad press, but the main point is that the saunas donated by Cruise worked. Some of the bad press had to do with the heavy niacin doses, which were part of the Rundown program.

Some of the personnel on Cruise's program experienced good results. A few of them even reported to have poured blue sweat when beginning the program. This was identified as manganese, a heavy metal used in some of the structures of the World Trade Center.

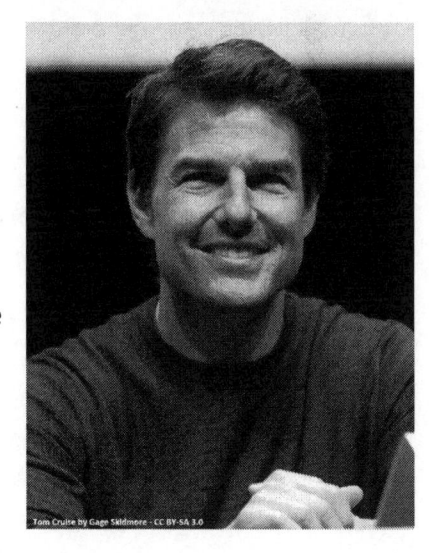

Tom Cruise by Gage Skidmore - CC BY-SA 3.0

Good press

Many studies exist in medical literature that underline the value of sweating as a form of detox.

In a 2012 study researchers identified 24 studies that looked at the detoxification effects of saunas.[37] Using these as a base, they found that there was real value in sweating. The studies showed that high levels of heavy metals were excreted in the sweat of sauna users, sometimes even surpassing the levels in urine.

Give it a whirl

It does not matter if you start with the steam room or the sauna, you owe it to your psoriasis to give it a try. Besides the various public or private facilities, there are many home sauna systems available. Unlike the old days when you needed to build a special room, there are new infrared-based units available that can be ordered online and then self-installed. Infrared units plug into conventional power points and can even be purchased as single-user units, which take up minimal space.

Stress apps

There are a number of de-stress apps available for your smartphone. Google some apps to try. When you use them at night make sure that your phone has a blue light remover app on it as well.

Inner balance

This app uses your smartphone and an external sensor that clips onto your earlobe. It helps you to monitor your moods and adjust your reaction to stress. You can also use it to track your progress, add notes and share your results. The app can be downloaded to your smartphone or tablet from the App Store or Google Play. It can also be purchased directly from the manufacturer HeartMath.

GPS for the soul

This app is from the Huffington Post and works without an external sensor (iPhone only). It's available in iOS and Android and can be downloaded from the App Store and Google Play.

ACTIVITY: The Third Horseman

Almost any kind of exercise will do you good. In fact, getting involved in some kind of daily movement is crucial for healing your psoriasis.

Before engaging in any purposeful exercise, recognize that standing is the most important daily activity you can engage in.

I know that psoriasis gets in the way of some activities, like swimming, where appearing in a costume is not a welcome option for some. But avoid the excuses and think hard. There are so many ways that you can be active that you must be able to find an activity that suits you.

Depending on your physical capabilities, walking is usually the best choice for getting started and you can read more about this in the chapter on walking.

Are you inactive?

If you are, then you have an opportunity to make a significant difference to your health. If you are active irregularly, then you can work to make exercising a few times a week a part of your regular routine.

You don't have to run a marathon, cycle 100 miles or build big muscles. Just get active!

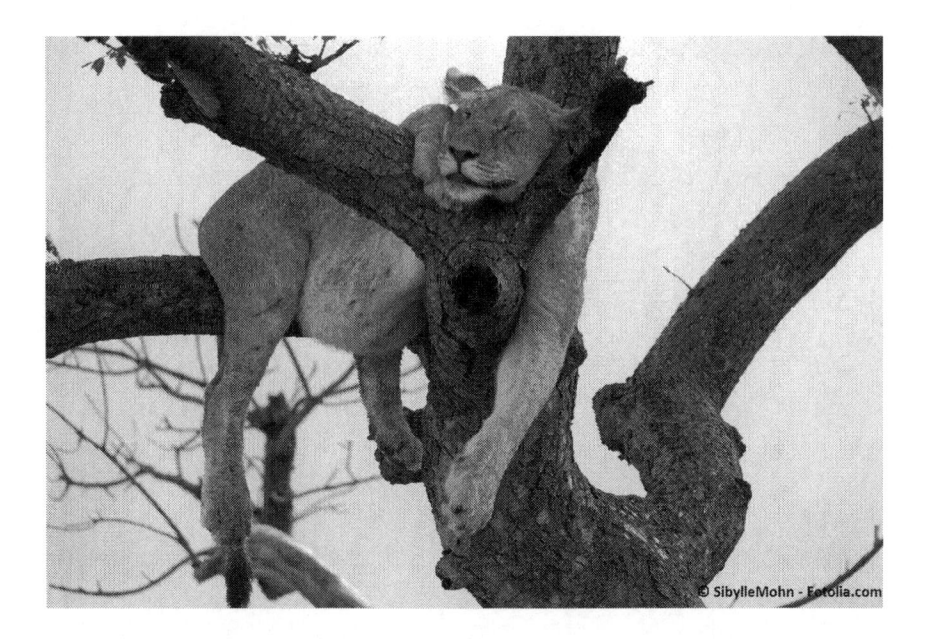

Effects of inactivity

Besides the negative effects on your psoriasis, these are some other dangers of being inactive:

- Heart and blood pressure issues
- Brittle bones
- Obesity
- Diabetes
- Increased risk of cancer, particularly breast and colon cancer
- Depression

Types of activity

There are many different ways to move or exercise your body. For the purposes of this book, I define two types: aerobic and resistance exercise.

Aerobic exercise is the type of activity you can do for long periods. Resistance exercise is any kind of activity that moves against weight, which can include moving your own body weight as well as making use of various kinds of equipment. We will discuss these in more detail in the coming chapters.

'I don't have the time'

Yeah right! That's the standard song that most exercise avoiders sing. If something is important to you, you will find the time and I can assure you that activity is important to you.

If you are creative with your time management, you will find a way to make the time. Some of my patients insist that they cannot make time during the week, to which I reply 'And what about the weekends?' That leaves the lowest common denominator at two days a week minimum for almost everyone.

Make a plan! The easiest way to remain consistent and committed is to design a customized program that works for you.

Your weekly activity plan

If you don't already have a weekly activity program, it's probably best for you to try out some options and then to see what works for you. From this, you will eventually settle on a weekly plan that you can stick to. Your plan should include some aerobic training mixed with some resistance training (weights), such as a walking or jogging day, followed by a day where you train against some kind of resistance. This is the kind of balanced program that most exercise specialists say works best to promote overall health.

It's important, but not life or death

Balance is critical. Yes, your program is important, but be careful not to turn any day in your activity plan into a life or death event. Missing a day's training may be unavoidable. When this happens, let it go because in the long term, a missed day is of no consequence and is not worth stressing about.

Stand up!

I believe that movement is non-negotiable. Irrespective of your physical circumstances and as long as you are not bed-ridden, you have to move your body.

Sitting is dangerous

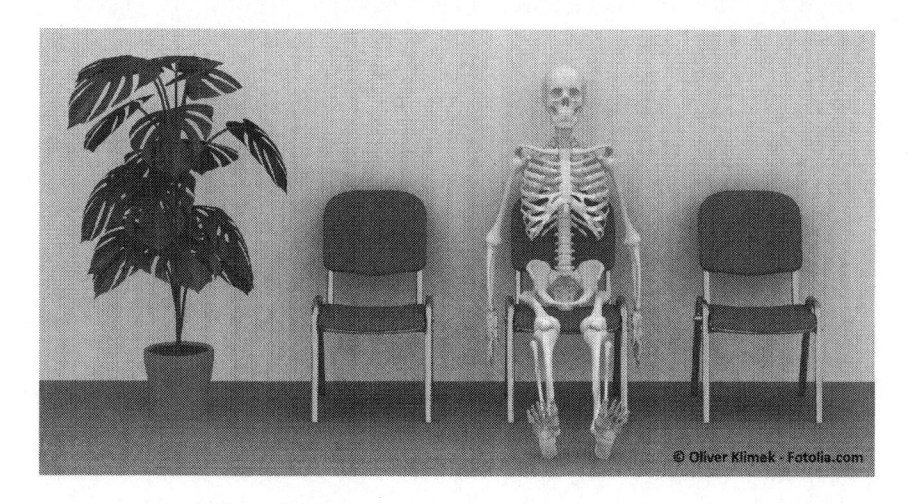

Your sitting habits need to appear on page one of your activity plan. Extended periods of sitting at your desk working or spending long hours lounging on your sofa are bad for your health. Research tells us that office workers spend an average of ten hours a days perched on their butts.[38] Working out for an hour a day does not completely mitigate the risks of spending the rest of the day sitting.

The longer you sit, the worse it is for your health. The World Health Organization recognizes inactivity as the fourth largest cause of death among adults worldwide. A pile of medical studies underscores why this happens. Lack of movement affects your health in many ways, including the fostering of a leaky gut and an increase in stress levels.

Sitting is the new smoking

Sitting is one of the most dangerous activities of daily life. A key comparison between sitting and the weightlessness experienced by astronauts was made by Dr Joan Vernikos during her time at NASA. She confirmed that astronauts aged about 10 times faster when weightless compared with the time they spent under the earth's gravity. She then went on to connect the effects of weightlessness to similar but less dramatic effects of prolonged sitting.

Be conscious of this risk and don't sit for too long. Fixing this is easy. All you have to do is to stand up once every 15 to 20 minutes. Nothing else is required. You don't have to run up and down flights of stairs, jog on the spot or do squats.

Just stand up! You can stretch or walk around your desk if you want, but that is all that is necessary. A recent medical study showed that standing three times an hour is better than 30 minutes in the gym. There are a number of timer apps that will allow you to set an alarm to remind you to stand up.

Exercise

I really want you to exercise regularly. It is vital for your health, your wellbeing and for the control of your psoriasis. For some people walking is enough exercise; for others running or gym sessions will do it. Even if you're desk-bound in an office all day, taking a 30 minute walk during lunch time will do you so much good.

Overdoing exercise = STRESS

Beware of over-exercising though; too much exercise causes stress and raises cortisol levels. Don't be one of those people who insert the phrase 'have to' into activities. I will always remember, after stopping for coffee with our cycling group after a hard 50-mile ride, the guy who refused to sit down with us because he 'HAD to do another 30 more miles'.

Seven activity tips

Before you start any activity, here are seven tips to make it easier.

1. **Don't exercise every day**. Rest as hard as you train. Your body cannot get stronger without having time to rest. Working too hard will hammer your immune system and make you more vulnerable to flu and other seasonal illnesses.

2. **Never miss more than a week**. Missing one or two sessions is OK but when you miss a whole week, getting yourself motivated to start again can be a problem. Don't let yourself fall into the 'I'll start next week' trap.

3. **Be inventive and flexible**. For example, if you are out of town and have nowhere to exercise, walk or run, find some stairs to climb or maybe even try a few guest sessions at a local gym. I was once in Norway where it was too cold to go out and my hotel lacked a gym, so I ran repeats up and down the hotel's emergency stairs.

4. **Listen to your body.** If you feel too tired to exercise, don't! Sometimes you can push through tiredness but if you are still tired 10 minutes after starting an activity session, give up and go home for a good rest.

5. **Never do two intense sessions in succession.** Always reward a hard day with an easy day. Too much intensity is bad for you. It lowers good hormone levels and raises levels of cortisol – the stress hormone.

6. **Don't spend too much time in the gym.** Some gym activities have the tendency to encourage obsessive behavior. Limit gym sessions to one hour on cardio days and no more than 40 minutes on resistance training days. In fact, I do my high intensity resistance session only once a week. It is really intense and never takes me more than 25 minutes, including the warm up time.

7. **Never worry about how you look when you exercise.** Some people I have exercised with came dressed to kill, wearing the latest kit and in some cases wearing makeup too. In the gym, there is no need to be self-conscious because no one will take any notice of you. Just throw on something comfortable and focus on what you're there to do.

Aerobic training

Also called 'cardio', aerobic is a fancy name for any kind of low- to middle-intensity exercise that does not cause you to get out of breath. My cycling coach explained it best: 'You're aerobic for as long as you can talk; when you start to gasp between words, you're out of the aerobic zone.'

Trained athletes can seemingly go forever doing aerobic exercise. Marathon runners run 100-milers and 24-hour events. The major triathlon events, most of which are heavily oversubscribed, have waiting lists of masochists champing at the bit to compete in an event comprised of a 4km swim, followed by a 180km bicycle ride, topped off with a 42km run.

Just because some humans can remain aerobically active for these types of efforts does not mean that it is good for you. A number of studies have highlighted the dangers of too much exercise. You need to strike a balance based on your capabilities, your level of motivation, and the time available to you.

Getting started

I suggest that you include one or two sessions of cardio training in your weekly schedule. If you are embarking on an exercise program for the first time or after a long break, start slowly. Less is better than more. I have seen many over-enthusiastic beginners go all out before they are ready, only to hurt themselves and then give up completely.

A gentle walking program is a good place to start (see page 114).

Consider a coach

Many beginners find the gym environment intimidating. Getting yourself a coach is a good way for you to get yourself into the gym with a professional to guide you. Your coach will also help you to set up a program that is tailored to your capabilities. Coaching can provide guidance that will ensure that you improve over time. Missing gym is much harder when you have a pre-booked session with a coach that you have committed to pay for. This kind of pressure will help to ensure that your exercise patterns become regular.

Lastly, don't get married to your coach. Once you have found your feet in the gym, consider going solo or even better, find yourself a training partner.

What not to do: Obsession

Once you get going, don't go crazy and become obsessive about timing yourself or competing with others. While a little competition is good, it is all too easy to become addicted to exercise and the competitiveness around it. Remember that you are exercising to be active, to improve your health and to lower your stress levels. Always, always enjoy what you're doing.

A case in point: I spoke to a competitive cyclist the other day about her rides in the Argus Cycle Tour. This is a race around the Cape Peninsula on what is arguably the most beautiful coastal road in the world. Guess what? After doing the race 18 times, she admitted that she had never once looked at the scenery.

My point is not that you should avoid competitive exercise. Rather, I urge you to avoid unnecessary goal-centric behavior if it makes you forget why you are doing it in the first place.

What not to do: Eat popcorn

The treadmills in my gym are super advanced and lack only one accessory – a popcorn holder. I say this because so many gym bunnies seem to spend their time on the machines watching TV or talking while moving at the pace of a tortoise. It turns the activity into a standing up movie experience, lacking only popcorn to munch.

When you do an activity, be there mentally. Try things like varying your pace, increasing and decreasing resistance levels to make your exercise more challenging and more engaging. Also, look at your form and try to improve the way that you do your exercise. Good form helps to ensure that you do not do repetitive movements that could injure you in the long term. Ask for some assistance or try to mimic the actions of someone who is visibly doing a more professional job of the exercise.

The staff walking around the gym are there to help you; don't be sacred to approach them.

Some equipment varieties to consider

The treadmill is the most popular piece of gym equipment. While most gyms have more treadmills than any other type of exercise equipment, there are many alternatives. Here are some of my recommendations:

Rowing machine: To me, rowing is the best all-round activity you can do in a gym. When done properly, rowing will give you a whole-body workout. It is also quite easy to vary the intensity of your workout as you row and hard rowing can make you breathless in minutes. The only downside is that to row properly requires some practice. Try to get a rower or a coach with some rowing experience to give you a lesson when you begin.

Elliptical walker: This can provide a good almost-total body workout when used with arm and leg movements. Because it supports body weight, it is often good for people with leg and knee issues. If you try hard, you can really tax your body on one of these.

Stationary bike: Great for any level or size of exerciser. Your setup on the bike is important, so get help when you start. Incorrect settings can lead to a painful ride or knee and hip injuries. If your butt hurts when you ride, get someone to check your setup. Discomfort quickly leads to the end of your time on the stationary bike.

Here is a list of some of the aerobic exercise activities you can do.

Outdoors:
- Walking or running
- Rowing
- Swimming
- Cycling
- Skiing

Indoors:
- Running/walking on a treadmill
- Stair climbing
- Rowing machine
- Stationary cycle
- Elliptical trainer
- Indoor swimming

Walking well

We come from a hundred thousand generations of walkers. Walking is built in to us because our ancestors walked and ran their whole lives. Today, we have little reason to walk. During the day we click mice, walking only to answer the call of nature. When we get home, we sit some more as we eat, swipe digital devices and watch TV. Machines move us around and we do everything we can to avoid moving.

If you start a walking program as a former couch potato, start small and don't set too many goals. Just walk a little and then rest. Be in the moment, enjoy the scenery, take notice of your surroundings. Don't focus internally on any aches and pains you might have. Don't give up; stick at it and try your best to get some joy from the activity. Over time, your distance and enjoyment will increase.

My Walk to Freedom

I started walking when I was 30kg overweight and couldn't climb a flight of steps without stopping to rest. I found that taking the first step was really hard for me and I procrastinated for weeks before taking my first walk around the block. My legs burned all the way and my aches and pains lasted for days. It took me a lot longer than I expected to get walking fit, and even longer for my body to start feeling the effects and benefits. Three years passed before I was able to walk distances without effort, but it was worth it in the end!

If you can, find a walking partner. Talking and walking together go well and your companion will keep you going when your motivation wanes. Do some research – there may be a walking group or club that you can join in your area.

Make walking your mission

Find innovative ways to increase the distance you walk daily. Here are some examples:

- Park further from your destination
- Walk wherever you can
- Use the stairs instead of the lift
- Get a step tracker and monitor how many steps you actually take every day. (Don't be surprised when you find out how little it is!)

High intensity walking

When you reach a stage of being able to walk regularly at a steady pace, you can enhance the benefits of your walking by adding some interval training to your walks. Doctor Hiroshi Nose of Shinshu University Medical School in Japan has tested the health benefits of interval walking versus steady pace walking. He split his test subjects into two groups. The interval group employed five cycles of fast, hard walking for three minutes followed by three minutes of strolling. The stroller group ambled along for the entire period. When tested three months later the stroller group showed almost no improvement in fitness levels, leg strength and blood pressure levels. The interval group, however, showed significant improvements in all these areas.[39]

The take-home message is: Don't stroll. Make sure that some parts of your walks are hard enough to cause you to become out of breath. Use Doctor Nose's method to structure your walks with intervals of hard and easy walking.

Resistance training

After walking, resistance training is the most important exercise you can do.

However, I find it hard to convince patients and the people I talk to that they need to do 'weights'. Many react with disbelief and often stop listening. Others, like my sauna companion, immediately come out with, 'I don't want to get big!'

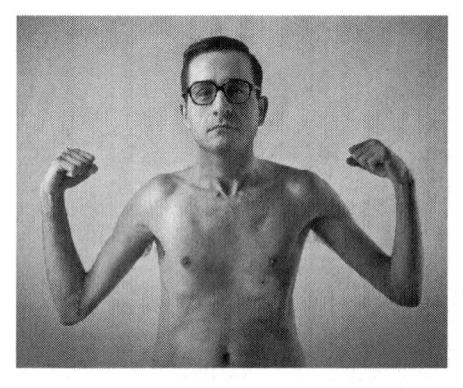

'Getting big' is part of the standard male lexicon, along with getting laid and getting rich. It has absolutely nothing to do with what we are trying to achieve. It also has nothing to do with stinky weight rooms peopled with tattooed musclemen. Believe me, these guys need to do things that are simply not normal to grow their muscles.

I think that training against some kind of weight is essential. Besides helping us to beat psoriasis, there are other good reasons to push weights. Two of the most important are:

- Weight training reduces the rate at which you age.
- Retaining or rebuilding your muscle mass is vital for your immune system.

There are a number of ways you can go about doing resistance training and I am doing my best to convince you to try it. I am sure that you will find a method that suits you.

Routines you can do at home

Body weight training

This kind of resistance exercise can be done pretty much anywhere. All these kinds of exercises are based on your own body weight.

Remember, as with any exercise routine, warm up first by walking or jogging lightly for five to ten minutes. Start any exercise slowly and work your way upward in terms of speed, the number of repetitions and the number of sets. Start with a single set and add more sets as you get stronger.

Here are some good ones to start with:

Squats: Stand straight with your feet shoulder-width apart, feet pointing slightly outward. Keeping your back straight and with your hands held out in front of you, slowly lower your butt, sinking down as low as you can. Keep your dips shallow at first, especially if your joints or leg muscles hurt.

Crunches: Lie face-up on the floor, knees raised and bent or if you are more comfortable, you can leave your feet on the ground. Put your hands behind your head or fold them over your chest. Slowly curl your head up towards your feet. Keep your neck as straight as possible; don't let your chin touch your chest. Squeeze your abdominal muscles when your head is as far forward as you can manage. Then release and uncurl gently backwards until your back touches the floor again.

Push-ups: Push-ups can be hard to do at first. If you find them too difficult, you can rest your lower body on your knees to make them easier. Lie face down on the floor while positioning your hands, palms down, in front of your shoulders. Push yourself upward with your hands. At the same time, breathe out and try to keep your body as straight as possible (don't curve your back). Lower yourself down until you touch the floor again. Keeping your hands closer to your body makes it easier.

Pull-ups: Ideally, you need a pull-up bar but often a door lintel will work just as well. To do a pull-up, stand beneath the bar with your feet together. Hold your hands up, palms forward, and reach for the bar. Keeping a tight grip on the bar, slowly bend your knees and allow your hands to take your full weight. Then slowly pull yourself upward. Once you are as high as you can get, lower yourself slowly again and repeat if you can. Pull-ups are hard so don't get discouraged. You can start by just hanging and then, over time, slowly lifting more and more of your body weight. Standing on a small box will also make it easier in the beginning.

You can use YouTube to source and watch professionals doing these routines. You will also be able to find other exercises that you may enjoy doing. Two YouTube videos that you can watch to get you started are:
- 10 Best Beginner Body Weight Workouts
- Bodyweight Exercises For Absolute Beginners

Gym routines

Weight machines and free weights

This kind of equipment is usually found in the depths of the weights section of your gym.

I am going to teach you a simple and safe high-intensity routine that I advise beginners and all people who push weights to use to get strong and healthy. The routine is derived from the work of Dr Doug McGuff, an Emergency Medicine physician with a passion for exercise science. Dr McGuff suggests that only a weekly single-set high intensity weight workout is required to build strength and maintain muscle mass.

Done properly, this routine takes about twenty minutes in the gym, including a warm-up.

The main aim is to work at high intensity and induce a deep level of muscle fatigue. This kind of short, sharp stress signals your system to grow and respond in a similar way to the effects of a 'fight or flight' situation. When you start doing this routine, any work you do will feel intense, so you need to increase the weights you use as you get more accustomed to it.

Five movements make up the main routine:
- A push away from the body
- A pull toward the body
- A pull down from the head to shoulder level
- A push upward above the head
- A leg extension

If you feel you can use more, you can add one or two more exercises, but sticking to just these five movements will net you 90% of your gains.

How it's done:
- The routine is designed to be done once a week or no more than once every five days (never do back-to-back high intensity days).
- Keep a note of the weight you use for each exercise. This is important, because it gives a progress history and serves as a reminder of how much resistance you need to set on each machine.
- Warm up using a weight light enough that you can do 20 repetitions. Get the feel of the movement. Load the resistance so that you can do a single set of between eight and twelve repetitions
- The slower you do the movement the better. Slower speeds almost entirely eliminate the potential for injury. Never jerk the weights.
- If you can only manage fewer than eight reps, your resistance is too high. Reduce the resistance.
- If you can do more than twelve reps, your resistance is too low. Increase the resistance.

The GOAL for each set is to go as hard as you can. Knowing that you have just a single set to do makes it easier to go all out. Failure to complete your last rep, no matter how hard you try, triggers an ancient metabolic mechanism that:
- Sucks glucose from your blood into your muscle cells
- Releases stored fat
- Increases insulin sensitivity
- Raises hormone levels, particularly growth hormone (HGH)
- Releases active substances called myokines that send positive signals to other parts of the body

You can learn more about Dr McGuff's research and his high intensity weight routine by Googling him.

Kettlebells

I'm a kettlebell fan. They are amazingly versatile and you can make a home weight room with two or three of them. Kettlebells originated in Russia a few hundred years ago and have been used for training in the Soviet army. They have recently become more popular and are used widely in gyms and homes today.

The ballistic movements you can do with a kettlebell build body strength and suppleness. Kettlebell movements mimic real-world movements better than static weight equipment. A kettlebell workout will strengthen your back, legs and shoulders. Go slowly if you have a bad back.

Start with a light bell while you get the hang of it. This also allows time for your muscles and joints to become accustomed to the work.

I think the best way to learn how to use kettlebells is by example. If you don't have access to an instructor, there is a selection of beginner workouts you can watch on YouTube.

Here are some good videos to get you started (search YouTube using the Video name):

- "Kettlebell Workout for Beginners – Invade London" (this is a fun one).
- "Kettlebell Workouts – Beginners Workout" (good all-round beginners routine).
- "Fitness Blender's Beginner Kettlebell Workout" (slightly more advanced).

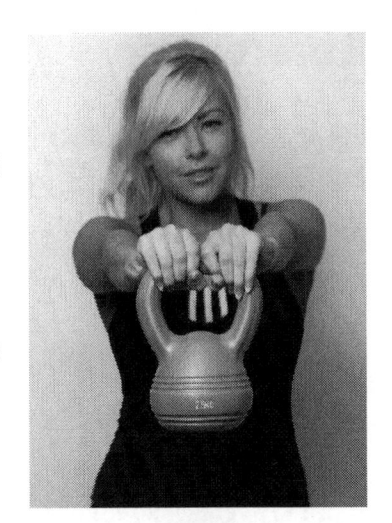

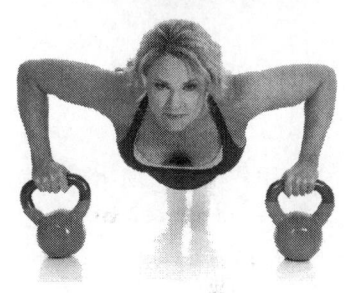

Body balance

In earlier chapters we addressed mental balance; now let's have a quick look at body balance. This is an extremely important yet never practiced skill.

As you age, your ability to balance declines. This translates into an increased potential for falls and spills. It is true that the older you are the harder you fall. So much so that falls are the leading cause of death in people older than 65.[40]

Your potential for falling will increase as you get more active so it makes sense to spend a little time every week working on your body balance.

Balancing methods

There are a number of ways in which you can go about strengthening your body balance. Here are the basic exercises you need to do. Once you have mastered these, you can increase the difficulty and improve your results by doing these same exercises on a Power Plate machine or using a stability ball or a half-sphere ball. You can also take up Pilates or yoga.

All the exercises below are done with a chair for safety. Once you become more confident, they can be done without the chair.

1. Single leg balance

- Place a chair within reaching distance in case you need to hold it to keep your balance
- Stand with your feet together and your arms at your sides
- Lift one leg and balance on the other

- Hold this pose for between 10 and 20 seconds
- Lower the leg and repeat for the other leg
- Repeat the exercise five or ten times

2. Clock balance

- Stand on your right leg with your hand on a chair placed on your right side
- Keep your head still and look straight ahead
- Hold your left hand out at the 12 o'clock position, directly in front of you, palm down and parallel to the floor
- Keeping your left leg as still as possible, with your outstretched arm parallel to the floor, sweep your arm to the three o'clock position
- Bring it back to the 12 o'clock position
- Then try and sweep it all the way back to your six o'clock, almost behind you
- Repeat these moves five to ten times
- Move the chair to your left side and repeat the exercise

3. Arm up and leg out

- Stand on your right leg with your hand on a chair placed on your right
- Keeping your body as straight as possible, raise your left arm
- Raise your left leg off the floor to the side of you
- Hold the position for 10 to 20 seconds
- Repeat five to ten times
- Move the chair to your left side and repeat the exercise

There are many more variations. Use YouTube to search for some examples.

My body un-balance

A while back, I was having coffee with some friends when one of them mentioned that his doctor had tested his ability to stand on one leg. 'Why on earth would she do that?' I asked. He didn't answer my question but simply said 'You try.' To my surprise and to the enjoyment of the group, I couldn't balance for more than a few seconds.

I resolved to become more balanced. The act of putting my shoes on became the daily tool I used. No longer did I put my shoes on while seated; I would only allow myself to do this standing up. It was initially a fiasco because I needed a wall behind me to balance against and so it took me much longer than usual. However, over the next few months it became easier and I can now do it quite easily.

Last week, while cleaning up around our patio, my foot became wedged between two objects, almost causing me to fall over. Without my improved balance I am certain that I would have fallen sideways and, with my foot trapped, broken my ankle.

The message here is that you should look at using simple strategies to slowly improve your balance.

Stretching and flexibility

While we are busy with the Activity Horseman, here is a short note on stretching and flexibility.

I don't think that it is necessary to stretch before every workout. In fact, some research indicates that stretching before an athletic performance (like running) may reduce performance levels. However, I believe that the additional flexibility that comes from well-designed stretching

ACTIVITY: THE THIRD HORSEMAN

routines is important for good health. These kinds of movements are designed to increase flexibility in areas important your daily life.

Being flexible has many benefits including:
- Preventing injuries caused by everyday tasks
- Improving your posture
- Enhancing your walking and running abilities
- Improving blood flow to your muscles

Be careful of trying too hard. Some stretches, especially those using motion to increase range, can flex joints beyond their range of natural motion and pull muscles and do damage to tendons.

Here are two YouTube beginner's stretching routines. Try them out!
- "Flexibility Stretches For Dancers, Cheerleaders & Gymnasts, Beginners Exercises Routine" (not that well named but well worth the watch).
- "Flexible in 5 Minutes: Daily Beginner Stretching Routine"

SLEEP: The Fourth Horseman

> *'...there will be sleeping enough in the grave....'*
> *Benjamin Franklin*[41]

The words of Benjamin Franklin capture our modern attitude to sleep. We admire people who work hard and sleep little. This kind of behavior seems to be a core trait of successful people.

Sleep is not wasted time

Unfortunately, we are wrong. Sleep is not wasted time. We cannot simply reduce our sleeping hours without cost to our health. Our bodies need sleep and our need for sleep remains the same as it has for millennia. We need our sleep as does every living organism on earth. Sleep cannot be deferred or 'caught-up' on like an overdraft can be.

If you don't sleep, you will die. This happens literally in a condition known as fatal familial insomnia, where increasing insomnia leads to death, usually in less than a year.

To fix your psoriasis, you need to sleep and, for many of us, sleeping properly is not easy. There are so many distractions and stresses that cause us to lose sleep. American adults, for example, get an average of 6.8 hours of sleep a night[42] and it's no wonder that almost 3% of Americans suffer from psoriasis.

Do the math. Assuming that you miss an hour of sleep a night, over a year that translates to 15 days of missed sleep! That's vital body repair time you cannot afford to miss out on. You need to aim for eight hours of sleep a night to support your other efforts to fix your psoriasis.

Dangers of sleeping too little

Advancing psoriasis, angry red patches marching across areas of pristine skin – that's the most significant effect of too little sleep.

A 2012 study clearly linked sleep loss with psoriasis flares, concluding that 'sleep loss should be considered a risk factor for the development of psoriasis'.[43] Lack of sleep damages your immune system and makes psoriasis worse.

Too little sleep also has other negative health effects, some of which include:
- Immune system impairment
- Increase in inflammation
- Reduced performance of general tasks (on days following a poor night's sleep)
- Increased risk of heart disease
- Development of a pre-diabetic state
- Diabetes
- Premature aging
- Increased risk of dying from any cause

A lack of sleep also affects you mentally by making you over-emotional and causing you to think more slowly.

Make sleep a priority

Charles Czeisler, a professor of sleep medicine, says that while Benjamin Franklin may be right about deferring sleep until death, 'not sleeping will get you there a lot quicker.'[44]

To fix your psoriasis and maintain your health, you must adopt a mindset that prioritizes sleep.

Your goal is to sleep 8 hours a day:
- Stick to a regular bedtime on weekdays and weekends (kids have bedtime and so should you).
- Develop a regular waking time on weekdays and weekends.
- Maintain a firm stance when it comes to avoiding activities that interfere with your sleep times.

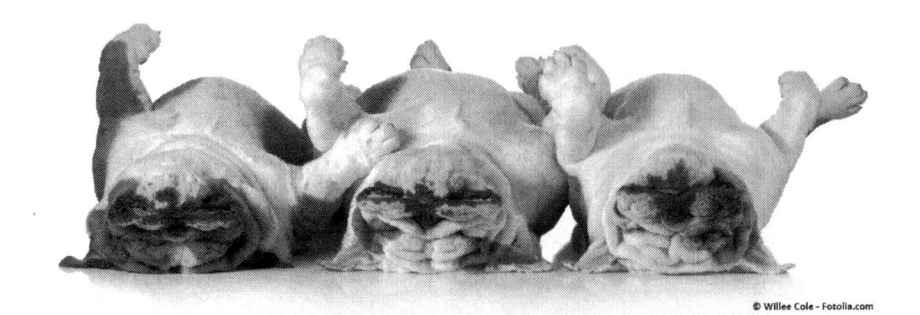

© Willee Cole - Fotolia.com

Enabling sleep

Many of my patients complain, 'Doc, I just can't get to sleep.' And to be fair we all have difficulty in getting to sleep at some time or another. There are ways for you to make it easier to sleep, without resorting to the use of sleeping medications.

While your sleep can be disturbed for many reasons, some beyond your control, there are some factors that you do have control over. You need

to make a concerted effort to manage these factors and construct the best possible sleep environment for yourself. Getting a dose of good sleep requires two ingredients:
- Good sleep-foreplay
- A sleep-enhancing environment

Sleep-foreplay

Why sleep-foreplay? I like the word foreplay for the ritual before you actually go to sleep because it is a necessary and integral part of the main event, which is getting to sleep. Similar to other kinds of foreplay, failure to prepare properly can radically affect the quality of the main event. Try to view the time before you go to sleep as a period of preparation with certain regular steps.

Switching off your TV and your lights and then rolling over and expecting to fall asleep is asking too much of your mind and your body. How can you expect to transition from an alert wakeful state to a sleeping state in a few minutes? You can't. Research shows that using an electronic device an hour before bed can delay sleep by over an hour.[45]

Your sleep foreplay should start at least an hour before bedtime. It will prepare your mind and body for the coming sleep event. Have a bath or a hot shower before bed to relax yourself. Light candles in the bathroom and add a tablespoon of Epsom Salts to your bath water. These will dissolve into your skin and relax you further.

Sleep enhancing environment

Regard your bedroom as a refuge, a place where you go to rest and recover. A refuge where the outside world has no place.

Your preparation should include:
- Removing all electronic devices, including TVs, tablets and smartphones.
- Dimming the light as much as possible. The dimmer the light before you go to bed the better you will sleep. (Read more about the effects of light.)
- Ensuring that your curtains block out all outside light.
- Covering any lights that may emanate from sources such as pilot lights or switches.
- Keeping the room cool (below 70°F/21°C); the warmer the room, the harder it will be to sleep through the night.

Electronic devices are a major issue and I believe that you should ban them from your bedroom. Do your TV watching and social networking in another room, before you go to sleep. There are apps that can control the kind of light emitted by your computer, tablet or smartphone.

You can also buy amber-colored glasses that you can wear at night to reduce the blue light falling on your eyes.

Other sleep-enhancing activities

There are things that you can do during the day that will enable you to sleep better at night.

- Reduce stress. Read the section on stress again. You must manage your stress to be able to enhance and increase you sleep.
- Get into bright sunlight (when you can); this helps to set your sleep clock.
- Do some exercise every day.

Light

Exposure to light, particularly blue light, will reduce your urge to sleep. Being in the dark will make you sleepy. As much as possible try to live like someone living without electricity. Follow the natural rhythm of day and night.

All this regular behavior came to a stop in 1879 when Edison demonstrated the first practical electrical light bulb at Menlo Park, New Jersey. Today, darkness is optional for most people yet it remains absolutely necessary to our health. Instead of becoming sleepy at night as the light dims, we are bathed in light from a variety of artificial sources. This light keeps us awake and allows us to extend daytime by many hours.

Even the eyes of the blind can 'see' this kind of light and blind people living in artificially lit environments adopt the same sleep patterns as the sighted people around them. This happens because their sightless eyes still absorb the light around them.[46]

What this means for your sleep

Now that you know that light keeps you awake and darkness makes you sleepy, you can use this knowledge to modify your behavior and your environment in order to sleep better.

Daylight

Most of us don't get sufficient exposure to bright sunlight. To sleep better at night, spend some time in bright sunlight whenever you can. Sunlight bathes your eyes in blue light which will help to set your wake/sleep clock and directly affects your ability to sleep better at night.

Get into the sun whenever you can. Aim for 20 to 60 minutes a day of direct sunlight. Spend your lunch hour outdoors if possible. Make an effort to be outdoors as often as you can; it will help you sleep and lower your stress levels.

Strategies for avoiding light at night

At night you need to reduce your exposure to blue light, which will keep you awake. As discussed earlier, dimming the lights in your home helps. Switch off any lighting that you can. Dim bright lights by fitting dimmer switches where possible and either remove bright light bulbs or replace them with dimmer alternatives.

TVs, tablets, cell phones and computers emit blue light and are major sleep-stealing culprits. There is a well-known app for computers and some smartphones called f.lux, which auto-adjusts screens to reduce blue light emissions at night. This works really well and I strongly recommend that you install f.lux or a similar app on all devices that you use at night. There are a number of similar apps for other makes of smartphones, like Twilight or Lux Auto Brightness for Android.

Melatonin

Melatonin is a hormone that helps to regulate sleep. It is also involved in other important functions including the regulation of blood pressure.

You can help normalize your melatonin levels by regulating your light exposure, which lowers melatonin levels during the day and keeps you awake in daylight. As it gets dark melatonin levels rise, making you sleepy and preparing your brain for sleep. This system worked perfectly for hundreds of thousands of years until Edison gave us the light bulb. Since then, our ability to light our night environment has drastically curtailed our available sleeping hours. Our use of evening light has messed up a mechanism that worked perfectly for our ancestors for over 100,000 generations.

Why is melatonin so important? To start with, it regulates your sleep patterns but it is also involved in gut health, bowel motions and it affects mood and stress levels. Regulating your melatonin levels will help you in many ways.

Regulating your melatonin levels

Blue light suppresses melatonin. The level of suppression is proportional to the intensity of the light and to the exposure time. So your takeaway from this is: Dim your lights at night and spend as little time as possible in brightly-lit surroundings.

Melatonin is made from serotonin, the 'feel good' hormone. Raising your serotonin levels makes you happy, while raising your melatonin levels makes you sleepy. Anti-depressants raise serotonin levels and thus reduce anxiety, improve mood and lift depression. Some of these are household names like vitamin P (Prozac), Zoloft, Celexa and Paxil.

You get happy when you sleep properly. This is because a regular sleep/wake cycle will naturally increase your levels of serotonin and melatonin, which boost your health and your outlook on life immensely.

Remember that if you have difficulty falling asleep at night, one of the causes is probably your exposure to light in the evenings before your bedtime.

Melatonin supplements

A melatonin supplement is not a sleeping pill; it simply signals your body to prepare for sleep. It is also a hormone and taking high doses can have consequences. Melatonin is used to treat sleep-related conditions like insomnia and jet lag. Doctors sometimes use melatonin supplements to treat depression-related disorders.

In the right circumstances, taking a melatonin supplement will make you feel drowsy and will help you to fall asleep. There are two different types of supplements: single dose and timed release. Some specialists believe that a slow release of melatonin during the night prolongs sleep. Try this only after you have some experience using the normal release kind.

Important: A short course of melatonin can help to regulate your sleeping patterns but long-term use is harmful to your health. Long-term use also has negative effects on the gut lining, which you definitely need to avoid.

Things to bear in mind when you take a melatonin supplement:
- Dosage is critical. Less is better than more. Most supplements are between three and five milligrams (mg), which is too much to start with. Break a 3mg pill into four pieces if you have to. Don't start out taking a dose that is any higher than 1mg a night. In fact, try 0.5 mg to start with if you can.
- Timing is critical. Never take melatonin during the day. Take your supplement an hour before bedtime.
- The effect is only active for 30 minutes. This means that you need to get to sleep quickly, so you must make sure that you are in bed with the lights off and ready to leave for dreamland no more than an hour after you have taken the melatonin.
- Take your melatonin course only for short periods. While there is no fixed course duration, never think of it as a long-term treatment. I would suggest that you take a two or three week course and then stop.

If you wake up and then can't get back to sleep at night, there is a trick that you can try using melatonin, which I describe in the next chapter.

Getting back to sleep

I bet you have had some MOTN. Not in the way that it's tagged in Urban Dictionary as an acronym for 'milk running out of the nose'. In our less exotic context, it's something that happens to all us at some time or another.

Middle Of The Night (MOTN) insomnia is the most common type of insomnia. It affects more than one in three Americans, waking them on at least 3 nights a week.[47]

Waking up is not the problem; getting back to sleep is the issue. Many of us wake up and then simply cannot get back to sleep. One solution is to take a pill and of course big pharma, who would never miss an opportunity for a revenue stream, has a medication (Intermezzo), made specifically for MOTN.

I don't think that medication has any place in your sleep. While it can be difficult to break out of a long pattern of MOTN, with some patience it can be done naturally.

Before trying to find ways of getting back to sleep, consider some method of preventing the act of waking up in the first place. Here are some to consider:

Reasons for waking up

- Alcohol before bedtime. Limit your alcohol intake at nights and don't drink at all two hours before you go to bed as alcohol can cause MOTN.

- Pets on your bed. Pets can wake you in ways that may not be obvious, such as making movements, noises or smells. If you have MOTN, do yourself a favor and find your pet a spot on the floor.
- Acid reflux is a common cause of sleep disturbances. A different sleeping position may help. Try sleeping with your upper body elevated. Sometimes losing some weight can help.
- Medication and supplements. If you take these before bedtime, try to vary the time that you take them to see if this helps you to sleep better.
- Depression is a common cause of broken sleep. You may not feel depressed yet your depression may manifest as MOTN.
- Joint and arthritis pain can often cause MOTN. If you have this kind of pain, try taking your pain medication at night, closer to bedtime and see how this affects your sleep.

Noisy sleep environment. Noises can wake you; if this happens to you, try to find ways to reduce the noise if you can.

What to do once you're awake

Once your eyes have popped open in the middle of the night, what can you do about it? Here are some workable options that will definitely help:

- The first rule is: Don't switch on the light and don't move! Staying as still as possible in the dark will prevent your mind and body from getting those 'let's get up' signals.
- Stop watching the clock. Marking off the minutes only heightens the stress of not being able to get back to sleep.
- Try relaxing your body to help you fall asleep. Start by tensing and then relaxing your toes. Then tense and relax your ankles, and slowly work your way up your body. Feel each part become loose and heavy.

- Once you are relaxed, try to breathe as slowly and shallowly as you can (see more about Buteyko breathing in the section on Stress: Breathing control). Breathe as if you are not breathing; this will lower your heart rate and blood pressure, which in turn will relax you even more.
- Now fix your thoughts, which may still be racing. Meditate (if you know how) or else try counting down from 100 and as soon as a thought interrupts your count, stop counting and then start at 100 again. The counting has the amazing effect of preventing the mind from dwelling on repetitive thoughts.

Melatonin hack: This trick is worth trying occasionally if you can't get back to sleep using the natural methods above. Take a small dose (about 0.5mg) of sub-lingual melatonin, a special fast-acting formulation designed to be placed under the tongue for quick absorption. Because it reaches the blood stream quickly, it will deliver a burst of melatonin that will put you to sleep within 10 to 20 minutes.

If all else fails, read this book; it shouldn't take long for you to fall asleep again.

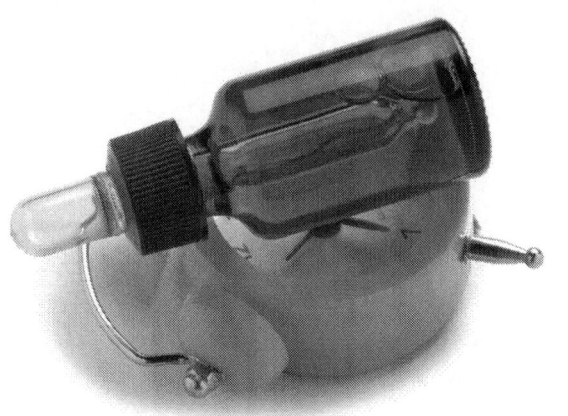

© Comugnero Silvana - Fotolia.com

A little MOTN prevention goes a long way

This type of sleeping difficulty can be caused or worsened by your behavior during the day.

These are some things you can do to improve the duration of your sleep:
- Avoid taking naps during the day.
- Don't fall asleep on the couch watching TV.
- Don't eat two or three hours before bed.
- Get rid of your sleeping pills. All they really do is put you to sleep more quickly, but the payback is that they do nothing for the quality or duration of your sleep.
- Recent anecdotal evidence shows that intermittent fasting can improve sleep.

Sleep apps

There are various apps for computers, tablets and smartphones designed to help you have a good night's sleep. They are useful if you are struggling to get to sleep, and some can also be used to monitor and document your sleep hours. Some of these apps are free and others are available at a small cost.

If you often use your computer or smartphone at night, seriously look at using a screen color adjuster.

Sleep enablers

These apps use gentle sounds, poems and music to relax you in bed and then hopefully send you off to dreamland. Unless otherwise stated, apps are for both Android and iPhone.
- "Relax & Sleep" by Glenn Harrold
- "Sleep Genius"

- "Yoga for Insomnia" (iTunes)
- "Deep Sleep with Andrew Johnson"
- "Insomnia Cure – Sleep Now – with Max Kirsten" (iTunes)
- "Free Relaxing Nature Scenes to Reduce Stress & Anxiety" (iTunes)

Screen color adjusters

These types of programs leverage our knowledge that blue light lowers melatonin levels. They hook into your local time and thus know when it gets dark. As soon as it does, they re-program your display to bathe you in an amber glow, which stops it from emitting blue light.

This works brilliantly and you will quickly get used to the soothing color of your new sleep-friendly monitor. I think this is a vital app for people who spend a lot of time on their computers, tablets or smartphones. It certainly works for me.

The best known app that does this is f.lux, which runs on Windows, Mac, LINUX and iPhone/iPad. There are also others on the market, so look around for an app that runs on your devices.

Sleep trackers

Rather than help you get to sleep, sleep trackers measure your heart and respiration rates as you sleep. By combining these readings with sleep time, periods of restlessness and sleep cycles, they provide insightful analysis with a sleep time log. Most sleep-tracking apps work in conjunction with a skin sensor that connects to your smartphone. Sensors are often wristbands but there are some under-sheet models. Some of these apps also include a wake-up function.
- "Jawbone Up" (wrist sensor)
- "FitBit" (wrist and other wearable sensors)
- "Beddit" (under-sheet)

- "SleepTime" (no sensor – uses built-in motion tracker)
- "SleepBot" (no sensor – uses built-in motion tracker)

Sleep-enders to wake up with

Amazingly, there are even sleep apps that wake you up! Based on the assumption that awakening during light sleep feels like waking up naturally, these devices wait until you are in a light sleep cycle before they wake you.

Skin care

In concert with an improved diet, reduced stress, regular activity and better sleeping habits, there are some changes you can make to help your skin heal faster.

The skin care chapter of this book provides a treatment plan and support to hasten the healing of your skin. This chapter includes information about:

1. GlyMag: A skin care treatment
2. Glycerin – humble wonder
3. Magnesium oil
4. GlyMag: How-to (step-by-step treatement guide)
5. General skin care advice for psoriatics.
6. Fighting a sudden psoriasis flare-up.

GlyMag: A skin care treatment

If you spend some time online trawling the various psoriasis community websites you will soon realize that they are awash with stories of miracle treatments that work for a few but not for everyone.

Over the years, I have done some patient online digging, reading reams of personal reports of psoriasis self-treatments. I have found that anecdotes with good news about the use of glycerin and magnesium oil appear consistently. However, I could find no reports describing the use of both together and over time. I have designed a skin treatment that combines them both, thereby offering the best of both worlds.

My GlyMag skin treatment uses both agents in a way that optimizes their lesion-healing capabilities, while at the same time minimizing their less desirable properties. Before I go into my GlyMag skin care treatment, let's take a look at the two main ingredients of the treatment, **glycerin** and **magnesium oil**.

Glycerin – humble wonder

Pure glycerin (glycerol) is a widely available colorless, odorless liquid. It is a naturally-occurring substance found in certain plants and animal fat, and it can also be made synthetically.

This humble, low cost liquid may well be the best-kept psoriasis skin care treatment secret! I urge you to try it out for a month or two; you may be surprised at how effective it can be.

It has two major benefits for psoriasis sufferers:

1. First, glycerol combines with a skin phospholipid (phospholipase D) to form a substance (phosphatidylglycerol) that affects the maturation rate of skin cells. If that sounds complex, the simple story is that psoriasis is caused by skin cells that mature too quickly and glycerin can help to slow this maturation process down. This gives glycerin the potential to slow or reverse skin plaques.

2. Second, glycerol is a humectant, which means that it attracts water into the skin. Higher water concentrations make skin softer and smoother, which takes care of dry skin, another area of concern for psoriasis.

SKIN CARE

Together these two features should make glycerin your first stop in skin care. However, there's more; glycerin may reduce itching and increase skin barrier barrier function.

Research into the therapeutic use of glycerin (glycerol) is sparse, probably because researchers have difficulty soliciting research funds for such a ubiquitous, low-cost item.

Dr Wendy Bollinger Bollag is one of the outstanding glycerol researchers. She and her associates at the Medical College of Georgia have published papers and applied for patents related to the use of glycerol. Their research has shown that the cell maturation effects of glycerol help to make skin look and function better.[48]

Researchers have also had good results with the use of glycerin in other skin diseases such as eczema.[49]

Buying glycerin

Purchase a good quality bottle of pure glycerin; it should only cost a few dollars. Look for a product that contains the fewest possible additives, colorants or fragrances.

Using glycerin

Use the glycerin undiluted if you can. If you find your skin turns red after applying the glycerin undiluted, you can dilute it with water. Try a 50:50 glycerin and water mixture and shake it vigorously for a few seconds. The water and glycerin mixture tends to separate over time, so always give the bottle a shake before applying.

Always be sure to massage the mixture into your skin thoroughly.

For the specific use of glycerine in the GlyMag skincare treatment, refer to page 145 of this book.

Magnesium oil

Magnesium oil is not really oil. It is a mixture of magnesium oxide and filtered or distilled water. The term 'magnesium oil' seems to be used by the natural health industry, largely because of the work of Dr Mark Sircus. He has written extensively about the medical value of magnesium oxide, which is often sold as 'magnesium oil'.

You can buy magnesium oil ready-mixed or you can make it yourself using a simple mixture of magnesium oxide flakes and filtered or distilled water. If you manage to obtain the magnesium oxide as a powder or as flakes, you can vary the quantity of water you use to adjust the potency of your mixture. Start by mixing one part of magnesium oxide to four parts of water. You can later increase the strength to 1:1, if your skin can tolerate it.

Ready-mixed magnesium oil is sold under various brand names, usually as a muscle and injury remedy. When choosing a 'sports' brand make sure it has as few additional ingredients as possible.

Magnesium oil:
- increases skin barrier function
- reduces skin cell proliferation (a key cause of psoriasis plaques)
- reduces inflammation.

Magnesium oil works wonders in reducing inflammation but it dries the skin and can cause it to flake. Glycerin reduces skin dryness and slows cell division (the core problem in psoriasis) but using it too often causes skin redness. GlyMag therapy uses both agents consecutively thus optimizing skin healing while reducing side effects.

I have had good results with this natural protocol. GlyMag is not a magic bullet that works for every case, but it works often enough for you to try it.

GlyMag: How-to

STEP 1: Start by applying the glycerin twice a day on its own for one week. Apply the glycerin undiluted by rubbing it into your skin lesions well. Glycerin works best when applied to warm, slightly damp skin. An ideal time to apply it is after your bath or shower. You can also apply it before or after a sauna or steam bath or when you are sitting in a warm or sunny area. Sweating seems to help absorption of the glycerin.

Note: Glycerin leaves the skin slightly sticky. Try to live with the stickiness for a few weeks; hopefully the improvement in your skin will make the discomfort worthwhile. Adding a thin layer of pure coconut oil on top of the glycerin does help to reduce the stickiness. You can also try using a commercial high concentration glycerin moisturizer like Yu-Be, which is more expensive but less sticky.

Watch your skin carefully for any adverse reactions.

Discontinue only if your skin reacts badly to the glycerin. If this happens, which is rare, stop the glycerin and move on to Step 2.

STEP 2: Now start applying the magnesium oil.

Since you should be applying glycerin directly after bathing, time your magnesium oil application to be at the opposite end of your day. For example, if you bathe in the evenings apply your magnesium oil in the mornings after waking. As with the glycerin, rub the oil thoroughly into your skin; use extra magnesium oil around painful joints and don't be shy about applying it to a wider area.

Sometimes the magnesium oil will cause a burning sensation immediately after application. When this happens, wash it off with flowing water. Then dilute your magnesium oil 50:50 with filtered or distilled water and use this diluted mixture for a few days. You can then try it undiluted again.

Ideally, this treatment should show results within four to six weeks. Be patient and persistent; do not expect an instant miracle. Try not to miss days.

Some options

1. If the glycerin has started clearing your skin plaques and you are happy with your progress, you can opt to continue using it for longer than the first week.
2. If you find that one of the treatments causes skin irritation, discontinue it and proceed with the other.

Purchase a good quality bottle of pure glycerin; it should only cost a few dollars. Look for a product that contains the fewest possible additives, colorants or fragrances.

Use the glycerin undiluted if you can. If you find your skin turns red after applying the glycerin undiluted, you can dilute it with water. Try a 50:50 mixture; mix it in the water by shaking it vigorously for a few seconds. The water and glycerin mixture tends to separate over time, so always give the bottle a shake before applying.

Always be sure to massage the mixture in thoroughly.

General skin and nail care advice

Be careful of soaps and washes

Almost all commercial soaps, shower gels and the like are swimming in chemicals that can worsen or delay the healing of your psoriasis.

Go NOW to your bathroom and throw out your commercial soap, body wash or hand cleaner. Then go out and buy some **glycerin-based soap** and use ONLY that soap from now on.

SKIN CARE

Protect your skin

Always think carefully before exposing your skin to unnecessary risks. As any experienced psoriasis sufferer knows, a minor skin injury can sometimes turn into a new skin plaque that will endure for years after the initial injury has healed.

Sunburn is a good example. Getting into the sun is necessary but excess sun burns the skin and can worsen your psoriasis. Use gloves when you are working with your hands. When using glues and other chemicals, be sure that they do not come into contact with bare skin.

Avoid anti-bacterial soaps

It is obviously important for you to wash your hands, since it lowers the bacteria count on your skin and reduces your chances of catching a cold or getting sick. However, using an anti-bacterial soap is overkill and potentially damaging to psoriatic skin.

Avoid anti-bacterial soaps like the plague. In the first place, they have been shown to increase infections rather than to decrease them. Secondly, they contain chemicals that can damage skin cells. Triclosan, an antibacterial that is used in skin and mouth washes, is one of these chemicals. It has been conclusively linked to cell death and has no place in the care of your skin.[50] Triclosan also accumulates in body fat and has been detected in mother's milk and in urine samples in as many as 75% of Americans over age six, where were tested.

Moisturize your skin

Dry skin attracts psoriasis plaques and you should be mildly obsessive about keeping your skin soft. Please read the section on Glycerin if you have not already done so.

Use magnesium baths and footbaths

Magnesium oxide flakes can be added to your bath water. This will help your psoriasis, relax your body and make you sleep better. Start using about a cupful of flakes. You can also use off-the-shelf magnesium bath flakes, which may have added fragrances to enhance your bathing experience.

If you are a 'shower person', you can make yourself a magnesium footbath with some warm water. Leave your feet in the water for 20 to 30 minutes for best results.

Nail psoriasis

Try making a warm magnesium footbath or a hand bath to soak your nails in. Try to keep your nails immersed in the liquid for at least 15 minutes. Use once or twice a day for a few weeks; the results may surprise you!

Fighting a flare-up

Sometimes your skin just gets worse. It starts to get redder and angrier with plaques that stand out like little mountains of misery. Sometimes there's a reason, such as a week of mega-stress, but often there is no definite cause. Reason or no reason, sometimes your psoriasis just takes off.

The question is: what can you do, besides taking some prescription meds, to slow down the flare-up and get your skin under control again? I don't have all the answers but I do have some suggestions:

Gut:
- Make sure that you are not constipated or even semi-constipated. Ensure that you poop twice a day. If needs be, increase your dosage of psyllium husks by taking it more often.
- Drink slippery elm tea every morning on an empty stomach.

Supplements:
- Up your dose of omega-3s. If you are taking flax oil, increase the dose to two tablespoons twice a day. (I sometimes add a couple of omega-3 fish oil capsules at midday as well.)
- Keep your vitamin D intake at 5,000IU or more daily.

Skin:
- As discussed in more detail in the earlier section on Skin care, the application of glycerin and magnesium oil can greatly help your skin.

Sleep:
- Make sure you are getting your 8 hours a day of quality sleep.

Sun:
- Spend some time in the sun if you can.

Stress:
- Take extra measures to reduce and manage stress (re-read the Stress section!)
- Exercise daily.

WHY

More about psoriasis

Psoriasis is usually recognized as a skin disease but it can also affect the joints and cardiovascular system. The involvement of organs besides the skin makes psoriasis much more than a simple skin disease.

> "Therefore, psoriasis could be viewed as a systemic inflammatory disease that increases vascular inflammation leading to MI and stroke."
>
> Medscape Article[85]

Usually starting as an eruption on the elbows, knees, back and scalp, psoriasis can occur almost anywhere on the skin. Psoriasis is also common in the nails of the hands and feet.

Skin affected by psoriasis has patches of raised, red welts covered by scales that often have a silvery sheen. While psoriasis can look similar to eczema, it usually affects the outer surfaces of the joints, whereas eczema affects inner joint surfaces and creases.

The name psoriasis derives from the Greek word for itchy; a feature that sometimes accompanies the disease. To me, the sound of its name is almost as ugly the condition itself.

Types of psoriasis

There are several types of skin psoriasis. Plaque psoriasis is the most common form and affects over 80% of all sufferers.
- Plaque (vulgaris)
- Guttate – the next most common type after plaque psoriasis; presents as small red dots and often occurs after strep (streptococcal) infections

- Pustular – small blisters filled with clear fluid
- Inverse – (flexural) occurs in skin creases and in the groin area (doesn't have scales like the plaque variety)
- Erythrodermic – distinguished by bright red skin covering wide areas of the body; may have fine scales

How skin psoriasis develops

Psoriasis causes skin cells to be produced too quickly. In normal skin, the average life span of a skin cell is about a month, but in psoriasis new skin cells are produced every four or five days. These new immature skin cells pile up on the surface of the skin, which becomes inflamed, painful and itchy.

Immune cells, called T cells, are specialized white blood cells designed to neutralize foreign substances as they find their way into the body. T cells are activated when they encounter foreign substances (antigens) like those found on the surfaces of bacteria or viruses. The T cell response activates a cascade of effects aimed at neutralizing any perceived threat.

In the case of psoriasis, T cells become confused and for reasons that are not fully understood, they migrate into the skin and initiate an immune response by releasing cytokines, which are small proteins used for cell signaling. Some of the cytokines released by the T cells cause accelerated skin cell production, while others initiate an inflammatory reaction. When this happens, the T cells attack the body itself, which is why psoriasis is classified as an autoimmune disease.

It seems that once the psoriatic process has begun, the damaged skin cells themselves release their own cytokines, activating further T cell attacks.[86]

Autoimmune disease?

Although psoriasis is widely acknowledged to be an autoimmune disease, some researchers believe it to be caused by a bacterial dysbiosis of the skin, which kicks-off the lesions associated with the disease.

A recent article in the publication *Experimental Dermatology*, has put forward the proposal that an abnormal response to bacteria in the skin may initiate psoriasis in genetically predisposed individuals.[87]

Triggers

Psoriasis usually erupts in individuals who satisfy these three criteria:
1. They have a genetic predisposition.
2. They have a leaky gut.
3. They experience severe emotional stress, a life-changing event, an infection (usually caused by streptococcal bacteria), or trauma from an accident, which triggers the disease.

Joints

Psoriasis is more than a skin condition. It painfully affects the joints of about 30% of all sufferers. The joint disease starts with mild swelling, which worsens over time and can progress to complete joint erosion.

A psoriatic joint becomes hot, swollen and painful to move. The disease affects the membranes inside the joints (synovium), causing them to thicken and become inflamed. The inflammation leads to expansion of the spaces between the joint spaces.

Joint involvement upgrades psoriasis into a systemic disease with bigger health risks. Conventional joint therapies usually involve drugs with non-trivial side-effects and pose long-term health risks to the patients who take them. Although usually an adult onset disease, psoriatic arthritis occurs in over 20% of all cases of juvenile arthritis

About 70% of patients who develop psoriatic arthritis present with skin eruptions before developing joint issues. To make matters worse for psoriatic arthritis patients, about 80% develop nail lesions. Psoriatic nails become thickened, yellow and pitted with painful areas of internal separation between the nail and the nail bed. It can take months for a nail lesion to grow out.

Cardiovascular risks

Psoriasis can affect almost any tissue in the body. I once read of a patient who had psoriasis in a heart valve! However, psoriasis is more commonly associated with increased inflammation in blood vessels as well as an increased risk of heart attacks. This blood vessel inflammation also leads to a build-up of (atherosclerotic) plaque in the blood vessels of the heart.[88]

A large Danish study found that psoriasis is associated with a significantly increased risk of 'adverse cardiovascular events and all-cause mortality.'[89] Overall, their figures showed a 54% increased likelihood of a stroke, combined with a 21% increase in heart attack risk.

Risks are highest in patients who present with the disease at a young age as well as in patients who have either severe skin disease or joint involvement.

Cancer

If the above list of issues is not enough, psoriasis is also associated with an increased risk of cancer, with cancers of the skin, prostate and blood (lymphoma) being the most common.

The gut

The gut explained

Since we discuss 'the gut' so often in this book, I have included a diagram showing its various parts, which you can refer to when necessary.

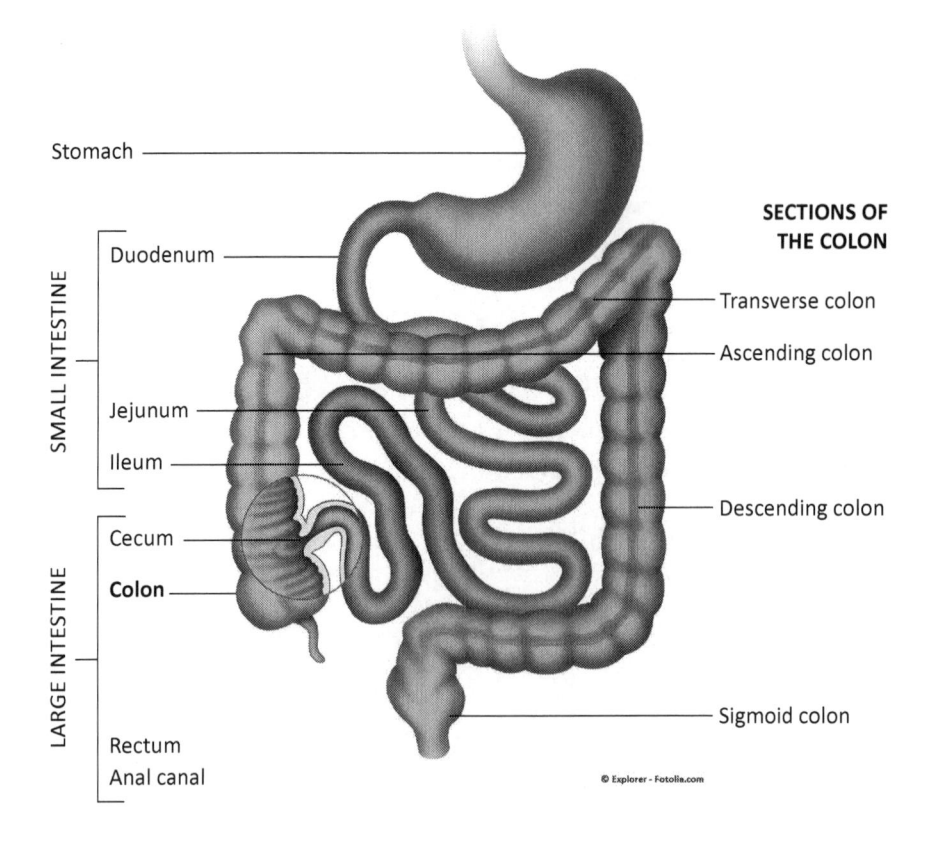

Pictured is the human gastro-intestinal tract showing all parts except the mouth. As we discussed in the section 'Re-imagining your gut', the opening of the mouth is joined to the exhaust at the anus in a continuous tube. The diameter of the tube widens and narrows depending on where you look along its length. It is at its widest when it forms the sack of the stomach and at its thinnest at the appendix.

Looking at the gut from the top to the bottom we see:

- **Esophagus**: starts at the top where it connects to the back of the mouth (not shown).

- **Stomach**: large gray bag-like area where digestion really starts.

- **Small intestine**: about seven meters in length and is made up of three areas: the duodenum, the jejunum and the ilium.

- **Duodenum**: a short C-shaped connector between the stomach and the small intestine. The duodenum is where bile from the gall bladder and digestive enzymes from the pancreas enter the small intestine.

- **Jejunum**: is around two meters long and has villi on its surface to absorb nutrients.

- **Ileum**: slightly longer than the jejunum. It is also covered in villi on its surface and absorbs digested nutrients that take longer to process. The ileum connects the small intestine to the large intestine via the ileocecal valve, which is shown within the circle on the left lower side of the diagram.

- **Large intestine**: is comprised of the cecum, colon, rectum and the anal canal.

- **Cecum**: a small area that is basically the entrance-hall of the colon.

- **Colon**: holds digested food contents from which water and other nutrients are removed, finally resulting in waste (poop), which is expelled. It is made up of four segments; the ascending, transverse and descending colons with the sigmoid colon at the end.
- **Ascending colon**: the area on the left of our diagram. Note that the colon has a wider diameter than the small intestine has and is far shorter.
- **Transverse colon**: crosses the body from the ascending colon (left) to the descending colon (right).
- **Descending colon**: the section descending on the right side of the body.
- **Sigmoid colon**: the area at the bottom of the diagram that includes the entrance to the anus; it is muscular and contracts to force poop into the rectum.

Leaky gut in more detail

Your gut is the largest point of contact between your body and the outside world. In your gut, all that stands between you and the outside world is a single layer of cells. These cells, called epithelial cells, make up the gut mucosa that guard the outside of your gut wall. The integrity of this barrier is crucial for your health and it often becomes damaged by the food that passes though.

If you look at the gut mucosa of the small intestine under a microscope you will see that the gut lining is covered with finger-like projections called villi. This is what they look like.

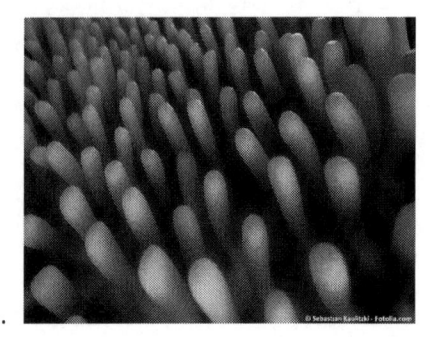

Each finger-like villus is covered by epithelial cells. This cover of cells over the villi is called the mucosal wall or 'the mucosa' for short.

Each epithelial cell starts its life in the crypts at the base of the villi fingers. A newly-made epithelial cell is forced to the top of the villus, which happens as a succession of new cells push it upward. Once at the top of the villus, the cell is shed off. This process is estimated to take about five days.

Having now seen the picture of real villi, here is a diagram that shows them as a magnified piece of gut wall.

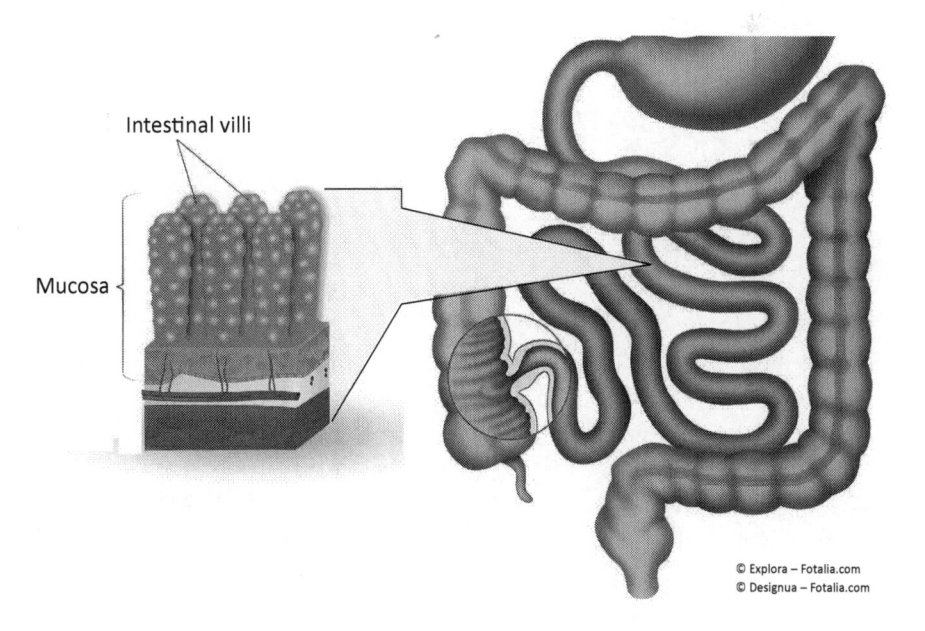

© Explora – Fotalia.com
© Designua – Fotalia.com

Villi

Now let's take a single villus finger and magnify it even more so that we can see the individual epithelial cells that cover the villus. The epithelial cells shown on the right in the diagram below have two important features. One of these is the 'little hairs', which grow on top of each epithelial cell. These hairs are called microvilli. In a living gut there is a thick layer of mucous layered on top of the microvilli. This mucous layer is critical to gut health and we'll take a look at it in a moment.

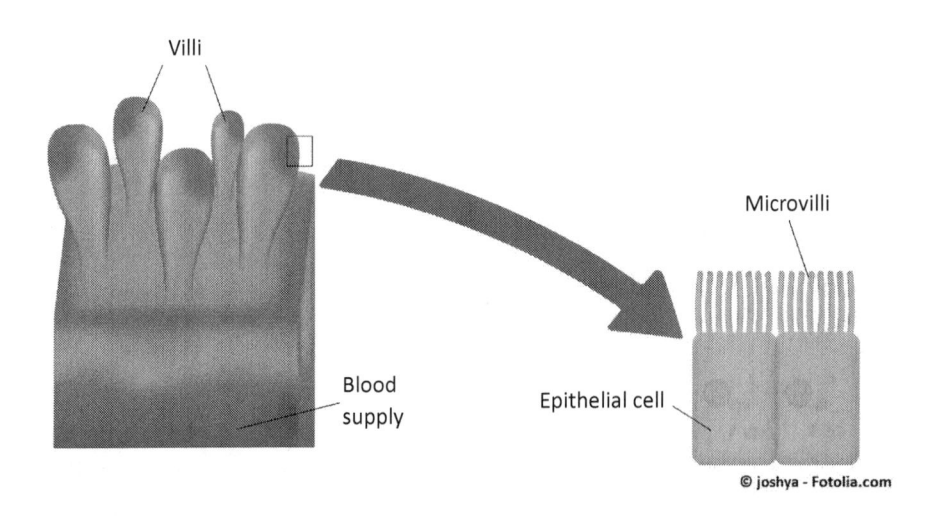

Villi

Microvilli

Blood supply

Epithelial cell

© joshya - Fotolia.com

Tight junctions

The other important feature is the area where the epithelial cells touch each other.

Each cell is 'glued' to its neighbor on either side by means of a complicated series of protein links. These links work like Velcro; they stick the cells tightly together and are called tight junctions. At present, about 50 different types of protein links have been identified.

One of the ways in which digested food particles get absorbed into our bloodstream is by passing through these tight links between the epithelial cells. Conceptually, when the tight junctions are closed, nothing can pass through them. They normally open under strict control, allowing various 'approved' molecules to reach the blood stream.

Some foods have components, like gluten, which force the tight junctions open. This allows molecules that would not normally be approved to cross into the blood stream. Once these types of foreign molecules are in the blood, they are attacked by the immune system and cause inflammation.

A pillar of this gut healing program is to restrict foods containing foreign components that cause tight junctions to leak, which then causes leaky gut. Sometimes exposure to these types of foreign substances stunts the villi and they become almost flat, like chopped-off fingers. This happens in celiac disease and severely compromises the ability of the gut to absorb vital nutrients.

Mucous layer

This is a layer of mucous that is tightly stuck to the epithelial cells lining the gut. This mucous is similar to, but not the same as, the mucous from a runny nose. The outer surface of this mucous layer is in direct contact with the food being digested. It is here in the outer layer of mucous that colonies of bacteria live.

These bacteria are of paramount importance to your health. Without them you would die. They process food, excrete substances that your body does not need and keep the growth of bad bacteria in check. When the wrong types of bacteria grow here your gut becomes damaged and you get sick. Most of the immune activity in the gut happens in this mucous layer.

This is a dynamic environment, which is directly influenced by the food you eat. This layer is constantly being rubbed off by the friction of food particles as they pass along the gut. Any part of the mucous layer that is dislodged is eventually passed in the poop.

Probiotics

When you eat probiotics, beneficial bacteria that have passed through the stomach can stick to this mucous layer and begin to grow a colony. As these beneficial colonies expand, they inhibit the growth of 'bad' colonies. This is why it is so important for you to eat fermented foods because they deliver the right kind of bacteria to your gut mucosa.

Prebiotics

Prebiotics nourish the gut mucosa in a different way. They are literally food for the bacteria and help good bacteria grow.

Into the toilet bowl darkly

Look back; I know it's not easy, but the remains in your toilet bowl tell stories. In fact, even how your poop hits the water, tells a story of its own.

Splashes

Not the most enjoyable topic but it's a good idea to interpret the splash as your poop drops. A healthy stool comes out in a fairly long sausage shape that is soft and normally glides into the water. When your stools hit the water like pellets or small stones, this is a sign of constipation. Of course, loose or wet stools indicate diarrhea.

Stool shapes

A good place to start is to compare your poop against the Bristol Stool Chart. Remember that you are aiming for a Type 4 on the Bristol chart.

Besides the various Bristol-like shapes, there are other aspects of poop that need to be looked at:

Diameter:

Beware of thin, pencil-thickness poop. If you have these, please discuss this immediately with your doctor. Overly-thick poop that can sometimes be too large to flush is also an indicator of a dietary problem. This kind of poop is often associated with an inability to properly absorb certain types of fat.

Color:

- Black stools can be a sign of bleeding in the gut. These kinds of stools often smell particularly offensive. Always report consistent black poop to your doctor.
- Bleeding, which you can see as a red color in the water, is often from hemorrhoids. If you see this often, discuss it with your doctor.
- Pale-color poop can be caused by medications or some antacids. If you are not taking these, it can indicate a problem in your gastrointestinal system and needs to be investigated by a medical professional.
- Yellow poop is not normal and needs to be discussed with your doctor.

The actual surface area of the small intestine

The surface area of the small intestine was previously thought to be about the size of a tennis court, but later research found the area to be a lot smaller – about the size of half a badminton court[4]. A standard badminton court surface area is about 82m^2 based on the official sizing of 13.4 by 6.1m[51].

However, researchers from the Sahlgrenska Academy in Goteborg Sweden have shown, using endoscopy on live subjects, that these long-used figures are incorrect. They suggest, instead, a figure of about 32m² for the area of the entire gut.

> **'The mean total mucosal surface of the digestive tract interior averages 32m², of which about 2m² refers to the large intestine.'**

This makes the small intestine surface area to be about one third of that previously claimed. Not a train smash but the original figure has been used as a benchmark in a multitude of books, papers and research articles. Don't believe everything you read in books, this one included!

The brain in the gut

The gut has a mind of its own called the 'enteric nervous system'. This makes the gut the only organ in the body that has its own nervous system. While the nerve cells in your head are concentrated in an organ called a brain, the nerves of the gut are widely distributed along the length of the gut – an estimated 200–500 million nerve cells – which is a lot more than that of a mouse (71 million) and at least the size of the brain of a rat (200 million).[52]

Lately, some scientists have taken to calling it 'the second brain' or the brain in the gut. This is because it acts by itself, separately from the brain, and can influence behavior.

This nervous system has a direct connection to the brain along which it sends and receives messages; this is called the vagus nerve. The nervous system of the gut responds to emotions and experiences. We have all experienced this gut-brain connection at times of great stress, or as 'butterflies' when we are nervous. Surprisingly, tests have shown that the gut sends far more information to the brain than the other way around. Poor health can send signals to the brain that result in depression, yet another reason for you to care about your gut health.

How your gut changes your mind

This means that the gut somehow dictates to the brain. Despite this deluge of information being transmitted from gut to brain, little of the information is perceived consciously. Conscious or not, these messages have real effects. Stimulation of the vagus nerve in depressives, who have been resistant to any other therapy, makes them feel better.[53]

With all this connectivity to the brain as well as its extensive body defense requirements, it is 'almost unthinkable that the gut is not playing a critical role in mind states,' says Emeran Mayer, Director of the Center for Neurobiology of Stress at the University of California, Los Angeles.[54]

In his review article, "Gut feelings: the emerging biology of gut–brain communication", Mayer explains that the gut and the brain are involved in complex bi-directional communications. He says that these communications result in 'multiple effects on affect, motivation and higher cognitive functions, including intuitive decision making'.[55]

Serotonin

The gut concentrates about 90% of the body's 'feel good' neurotransmitter, serotonin.

Frankly, other than its role in gut movement, we have no idea what serotonin does in the gut.[56] We know that serotonin is directly involved in balancing moods and that we can make someone happier by raising their serotonin levels. It is very much part of the successful functioning of popular mood-lifting drugs like Zoloft, and a host of others.

We also know of some of serotonin's actions beyond the gut. It is somehow involved in bone maintenance. Inhibiting its manufacture in the gut increases bone growth in the bones of rodents with osteoporosis (and no ovaries).[57]

Bacteria communicate with your brain!

It is becoming increasingly clear that the bacteria in our gut can affect our thinking in ways that were never considered before. This kind of communication goes way beyond the chain of events that occur after consuming a meal containing toxic bacteria that produces feelings of nausea and discomfort that we all experience from time to time.

Have you ever had one of those urgent, anxious sugar cravings? The kind where all self-restraint goes out the window and you end up scoffing mounds of sugar-laden foods, only to be drowned by waves of remorse a short while later? Would you believe that scientists are busy proving that some sugar cravings are initiated by gut bacteria? They think that hungry sugar-loving bacteria produce neuroactive chemicals that initiate signals from the enteric nervous system to the brain. These announce, in no uncertain terms, that you NEED SUGAR!

It is proof enough for me that sugar cravings disappear in many of my low-carb patients after a few weeks of no sugar. I am pretty sure that the lack of sugar kills off most of these sugar-loving bacteria and thus turns off the source of the sugar cravings.

Other researchers have been able to cause behavioral abnormalities associated with mental states like anxiety and autism in normal mice by injecting them with substances produced by gut bacteria.

We have a lot to learn in this area, but in the meantime, it is crystal clear that healing your gut will go a long way towards healing your mind and body.

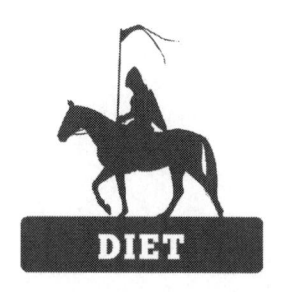

DIET: The First Horseman

More on reading nutrition facts labels

On the pages that follow, I present a series of nutrition facts labels from various products and I explain how to read them. I suggest that you go through the examples and try to spot the important (dangerous) ingredients.

You are most interested in:
1. Glycemic carbs (sugars) – the stuff we are trying to avoid
2. Portion size

Example: Full fat cream

If you can tolerate dairy, I recommend cream as a milk substitute. It has fewer carbs than milk, tastes better, and has the major benefit of making you feel full a whole lot quicker than milk does. If you have to have milk, make sure it is full cream and not a low fat variety that has substituted the wholesome fat for milk sugars instead. View the milk label overleaf.

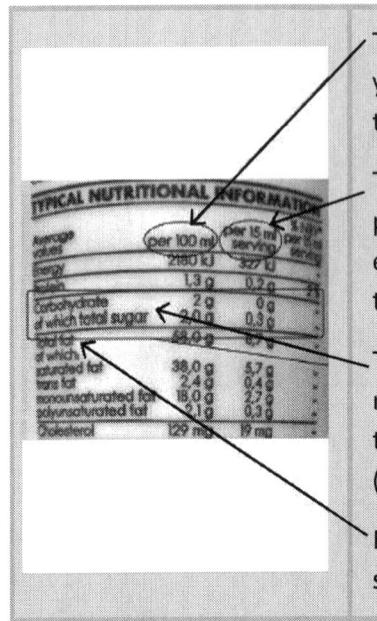

The 100ml column here is useless until you know the actual container size, in this case, 250ml.

The serving size of 15ml is an average portion size and you can usually estimate your carb load from values in this column.

These are the numbers that we are most interested in. We want to know total carbohydrates that are glycaemic (i.e. will cause insulin to rise).

Believe it or not, this cream is good stuff to eat!

Example: Balsamic vinegar

Balsamic vinegar is a common ingredient in salads and is viewed as a healthy choice. It may be, but be cautious as to how much of it you use. A quick read of the label below should alarm you enough to know that this particular brand needs to be used sparingly. (Since balsamic vinegar is made by double fermenting various fruits, the carb count will vary widely between brands; make sure you select a low carb variety.)

It may be surprising to find that balsamic vinegar contains a lot of carbs!

This balsamic vinegar has a lot of carbs! A tablespoon (15ml) will have almost 6g of carbs. Be careful to use only a small amount; a big splash of this stuff could ruin your whole day.

DIET: THE FIRST HORSEMAN

Example: Breakfast cereal

Remember that it is the glycemic carbs that affect your blood sugar levels. There is no prize for figuring out that this stuff will make you fat.

TYPICAL NUTRITIONAL INFORMATION		
Average Values	per 100 g	per 45 g serving
Energy	1518 kJ	683 kJ
Protein	12,4 g	5,6 g
Glycaemic carbohydrate	58 g	26 g
of which total sugar	10,6 g	4,8 g
Total fat	6,5 g	2,9 g
of which		

This breakfast cereal is hardly the breakfast of champions! One serving has 26g of carbs.

You would consume your entire day's allocation of carbs in one bowl!

Example: Sugar, the king of carbs

Sugar, as you may have realized by now, is the star of the show in terms of packing on weight and damaging your health.

> '... if only a small fraction of what is already known about the effects of sugar were to be revealed in relation to any other material used as a food additive, that material would promptly be banned.'
>
> *John Yudkin* – Pure White and Deadly

Note the conversion at the bottom of the image below from a sugar packet.

NUTRITIONAL INFORMATION		
Typical Values	per 100 g as packed	per 4 g serving (as packed)
Energy	1698 kJ	68 kJ
Protein	0 g	0 g
Glycaemic Carbohydrate	100 g	(4 g)
of which		
total sugar	100 g	4 g
Total Fat	0 g	0 g
of which		
saturated fat	0 g	0 g
trans fat	0 g	0 g
monounsaturated fat	0 g	0 g
polyunsaturated fat	0 g	0 g
Dietary Fibre	0 g	0 g

Nice glycaemic load here!

As a rule of thumb, 1 teaspoon of sugar equals almost 5g of carbs. Just imagine 7 teaspoons of this stuff in your Coke or 9 of them in your 'healthy' fruit juice.

Example: Maize (corn meal)

Maize is a cereal grain that is part of the staple diet of many people throughout the world.

It is America's largest crop and corn is grown on over 400,000 American farms.[58] A genetic variant is called Sweet Corn. Corn is high in carbs and contains very little fiber. Somewhere around 6% of America's corn crop is converted to High Fructose Corn Syrup and appears in many foodstuffs.

Corn is also problematic for psoriatics. It has many strange and new antigens that damage the gut and can trigger abnormal immune responses.

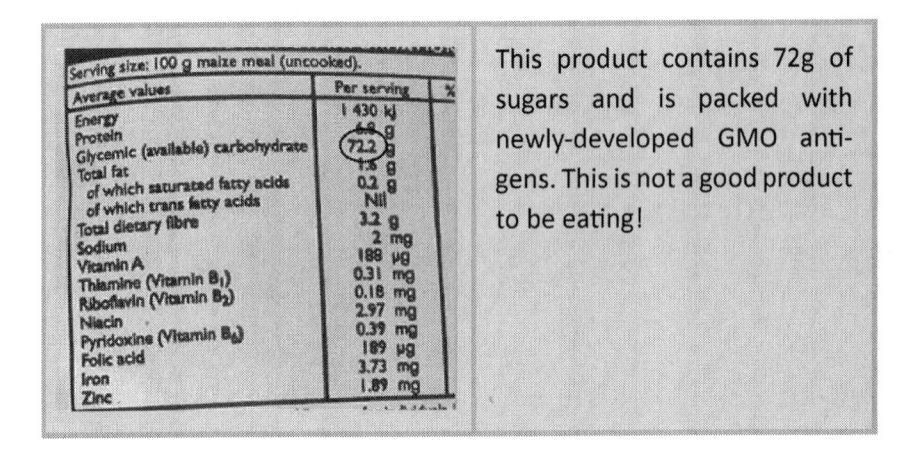

Serving size: 100 g maize meal (uncooked).		
Average values	Per serving	%
Energy	1 430 kJ	
Protein	6.6 g	
Glycemic (available) carbohydrate	72.2 g	
Total fat	1.5 g	
of which saturated fatty acids	0.2 g	
of which trans fatty acids	Nil	
Total dietary fibre	3.2 g	
Sodium	2 mg	
Vitamin A	188 µg	
Thiamine (Vitamin B₁)	0.31 mg	
Riboflavin (Vitamin B₂)	0.18 mg	
Niacin	2.97 mg	
Pyridoxine (Vitamin B₆)	0.39 mg	
Folic acid	189 µg	
Iron	3.73 mg	
Zinc	1.89 mg	

This product contains 72g of sugars and is packed with newly-developed GMO antigens. This is not a good product to be eating!

Corn and High Fructose Corn Syrup should be avoided at all costs.

Example: Whole-wheat pasta

Don't eat pasta as it delivers a double whammy for psoriatics. It is full of sugar and is made of wheat, probably the two most important foods for psoriasis suffers to avoid.

DIET: THE FIRST HORSEMAN

> **Pasta**
>
> Most pasta is about 70% pure carbs. Highly active and easy to digest, it quickly spikes blood sugar and since it is usually eaten in big bowlfuls, it is a danger to be avoided.

You can read the labels!

Practice and you will get better at it. If you find a label that is hard for you to decipher, take a pic and mail it to me. I would be happy to help. 4HorseMen@biohacks.guru

Why our modern diet is so bad

As humans, we were never designed to eat sugars in anything but tiny quantities. We did not eat grains in any appreciable quantity either, mainly because we lacked the fire to cook the grains into an edible form.

> 'Hunter-gatherers practiced the most successful and longest-lasting life style in human history. In contrast, we are still struggling with the mess into which agriculture has tumbled us, and it's unclear whether we can solve it.'
>
> Jared Diamond, The Worst Mistake in the History of the Human Race.[59]

We originated in a world where sugar was so rare that we became hardwired to seek out and consume as much sugar or sweet stuff as we could get our hands on. The call of 'sweet' is so strong that it even overrides other supposedly stronger addictions, like cocaine. A recent lab test proved this conclusively by making cocaine-addicted lab rats choose between sugar and their cocaine habit. Guess which they chose? They went for the sweet stuff, every time.[60]

You are also programmed to seek sweetness in a similar way to those lab rats. It is a powerful urge; be wary of it at all times.

200,000 years of practice

We humans have existed largely unchanged for two hundred thousand years or so. Over this period, our diet and activities remained unchanged. It is only in the past few thousand years, with the advent of agriculture, that our habits have been radically altered.

Today our bodies are faced with challenges from:
- Sweetness and global availability of high impact sugars
- Wheat, corn and other mass-produced agricultural products
- Pesticides
- Food additives

Besides the damage sugars cause, the presence of wheat in our diet also bombards our gut with an array of foreign substances. Gluten is the worst of these, but there are many others.

Missing stuff

Some vital nutrients that have been present in our food supply for millennia have vanished or changed in some profound way.

Omega-3 fats

Omega-3 fatty acids are just about absent from our modern food supply because omega-3s and shelf life are mutually exclusive. The higher the omega-3 content in a foodstuff, the faster it goes off. Thus almost all the food in your supermarket has had omega-3s removed to make it last longer. Remember the guy who found a perfectly-preserved burger in his coat pocket 14 years after he bought it? The burger still looked the same.[61] The reason? It contained no omega-3s.

One of the processes food manufacturers use to promote shelf life is to hydrogenate these omega-3 fatty acids, which turns them into bad fats. The process results in the terms 'partially hydrogenated' or 'hydrogenated' on food labels. Avoid any food products with these words in the ingredients.

There are three types of omega-3s that you need to supplement; ALA, EPA and DHA. Omega-3s are a critical supplement that will help balance the ratio of omega-6s and omega-3s in the tissues of your body. In general omega-6s are pro-inflammatory, while omega-3s reduce inflammation.

Ideally, at least 1 gram of EPA and DHA (combined) daily is recommended. EPA and DHA should be available in a diet rich in fish, but the most convenient way is to take an omega-3 supplement. Be careful with your supplement choice as there are many low-quality fish oils available out there. Rather pay a bit more for a brand that clearly states it contains no mercury or other contaminants.

Try to ensure that the EPA and DHA quantities in the capsule or tablet that you select add up to about 1 gram. Cheaper varieties often have reduced levels of these two vital ingredients.

By way of example, here are the contents of a single 1,000 mg capsule in my cupboard:

Concentrated Salmon Oil 1,000 mg:
- EPA – 198mg
- DHA – 132mg

You need three of these to get your recommended 1 gram (1,000mg) per day, i.e. 3 x 330mg (198 plus 132) per capsule.

Try and increase your intake of fish, especially salmon, sardines and other cold water fish, to boost your omega-3 intake.

Vitamin D

Almost all of us are deficient in vitamin D because we no longer spend much time in the sun. Vitamin D is so critical to our health that new health functions for it seem to pop-up every month. And sure enough, vitamin D is also vital for good gut health.

Supplements

L-Glutamine

Glutamine (or L-glutamine) is a conditionally essential amino acid. It is the most abundant amino acid in the blood. It can be manufactured in the body, mostly in muscle. Under stressful conditions such as illness and stress, it becomes essential.

Medical science has realized that glutamine is essential for gut health. For instance, it is now common practice to add glutamine to the drips of patients who cannot eat food by mouth.[62]

> **'Glutamine plays a key role in intestinal growth and maintenance of gut function'**[63]

Glutamine is essential for gut health. It is vital for the repair and maintenance of strong gut mucosa. Studies have shown that it protects against mucosal breakdown and promotes growth of new epithelial cells. It also supports immune functions in the gut.[64] Glutamine also acts to limit the growth of bad gut bacteria.

Take your glutamine every day! In the supplements section I advise a teaspoonful (5g) of L-glutamine once or twice daily in a glass of water.

Flax seed oil

I strongly suggest a tablespoon or two of good flax seed oil daily, in addition to your fish oil capsules.

It has high levels of ALA (alpha-linoleic acid) as well as moderate DHA and EPA levels. Always keep your opened flax seed oil bottle in the fridge.

Vitamin D

If I were allowed only one supplement, I would choose vitamin D.

An alarming number of people are deficient in vitamin D. Researchers have consistently found this to be the case in between 30 to 80% of the U.S. population. A 2011 study of 4,495 adult participants found that 82% of the black people in the study were vitamin D deficient.[65]

The reason for this is that few foods naturally contain vitamin D and people are spending less time in the sun. The widespread use of sunscreen preparations also reduces the skin's ability to make vitamin D.

Leaky gut

Low levels of vitamin D may increase gut permeability.

Get into the sun

Our modern 'sun phobia' is a situation where sun exposure has been demonized and has resulted in most people either avoiding the sun altogether or else wearing sunscreen whenever they are exposed to sunlight. To make matters worse, our clothes also limit our body's exposure to the sun.

Even in sunny climes, where natural maintenance of normal vitamin D levels would be possible, many avoid sun exposure and become deficient in this vital hormone.

What are the consequences of vitamin D deficiency? Here is a short list:
- Leaky gut tendencies
- Compromised immune functions
- Depression (especially seasonal)
- Increased susceptibility to breast cancer
- Weight gain and increased insulin resistance

Food supply

Dairy products and certain fatty fish contain vitamin D. In addition, many foods such as cereals and milks are fortified with vitamin D.

It is essential for your health and for the recovery of your psoriasis, that you spend some time in the sun as well as supplementing daily with vitamin D3.

Magnesium

At the core of the molecule that gives life to this planet is an atom of magnesium. The molecule is chlorophyll and it allows plants to capture energy from the sun and to store it in a chemical form. The ability for cells to use this stored energy is fundamental to all life.

Magnesium performs many vital body functions and to name a few, it is involved in:
- Energy production
- Muscle movement

- Calcium absorption
- Immune function
- Heart rhythm
- Blood pressure regulation
- Bone health
- Vitamin D metabolism
- DNA production and protection
- Neurotransmitters

Our modern diet has caused an epidemic of low magnesium levels and about 60 to 80% of people worldwide are estimated to be magnesium deficient. Psoriatics often have low blood levels of magnesium and vitamin D. One of the best known treatments for psoriasis is to spend a few weeks at the Dead Sea. It is not coincidental that the water of the Dead Sea has a high magnesium concentration. A 2005 study reported in the *International Journal of Dermatology* that the magnesium-rich salt of the Dead Sea improved skin barrier function and reduced inflammation in skin conditions like psoriasis.

Besides psoriasis there are some other conditions that show improvement from corrected magnesium levels:

- Osteoporosis – which is more likely to be caused by low magnesium levels rather than a lack of calcium as is popularly believed
- Hypertension – high blood pressure can be reduced when magnesium levels are normalized
- Type II diabetes
- Depression
- Arrhythmias (abnormal heart rhythms)
- Inflammation of blood vessels

Restoring your magnesium levels

Poor absorption from the gut is partly the cause of chronic low magnesium levels. Some of the factors that cause this are:

- Magnesium is absorbed with difficulty from digested food
- Loose stools and diarrhea occur as soon as magnesium levels in food supplements become too high
- Psoriatics may have a gene mediated reduction in the capacity to absorb magnesium from the gut

In addition to taking a magnesium supplement, the daily application of a magnesium chloride solution to the skin is an excellent way to deliver magnesium directly to affected areas and to increase blood magnesium levels. Various studies have shown an increase of blood levels of magnesium after a few weeks of transdermal application of magnesium chloride.

Use my GlyMag skin treatment to help heal your skin plaques and at the same time raise your magnesium levels.

Biotics: Pre-, pro- and post-

The various flavors of pre- and probiotics are all intended to correct imbalances in the types and quantities of bacterial colonies that grow in our gut. Postbiotics are produced by bacteria and have value to the bacteria themselves and to the body that hosts them.

For anyone who argues that prebiotics and probiotics are a 'health fad', here's a simple fact that will end the argument: Breast milk comes with both. Mother's milk contains both live bacteria and a sugar-based prebiotic (galacto-oligosaccharide).

Our modern sugar-laden diet promotes the growth of unfriendly and unhealthy bacteria in our gut. You can imagine this kind of imbalance as a garden that is not well tended and consequently becomes weed-infested. Importantly, continuing the weed analogy, removing weeds and re-growing good vegetation requires the right fertilizers, time and consistent work.

Successfully balancing and rejuvenating your gut bacteria will, in the same way as the garden, require time and consistency.

Prebiotics

Prebiotics are indigestible substances that aid or support the growth of the beneficial bacteria inside or on our bodies. The prebiotics available today almost exclusively target the organisms living inside our gut. However, recent developments point to a new area of skin prebiotics, with creams containing prebiotics specifically designed to nourish beneficial skin bacteria.

Most prebiotics are made from fiber that our systems cannot digest. The beneficial bacteria in our gut ferment these fibers to provide them with nourishment to help them grow. The bacteria that digest prebiotics are found in the colon (large intestine). Food normally passes through the small intestine too quickly for this kind of fermentation.

In general, prebiotics will aid the growth of bifido bacteria and lactobacilli, two groups of beneficial bacteria that enhance food digestion and boost immune functions.

The two major types of prebiotics are short-chain and long-chain. Short-chain prebiotics, the best-known of which is FOS (fructo-oligosaccharide), are fermented quickly because of their small molecular size. Because they ferment more quickly, short-chain prebiotics work mostly in the ascending colon. Longer-chain prebiotics like inulin and resistant starch provide nourishment to the bacteria in the transverse and descending colons.

Resistant starch: This is a 'special type' of carbohydrate that cannot be broken down into sugars during digestion. Resistant starch is found in foods like potatoes, pasta, beans and lentils. A good way to take resistant starch is in the form of potato starch, which you can mix with water. Bacteria in the large intestine can break resistant starch down into short-chain fatty acids such as butyrate.

Butyrate: One of the beneficial effects of eating prebiotic fibers is that they increase the concentration of butyric acid (butyrate) in the colon. This short-chain fatty acid has been studied in mice where it has been shown to increase heat production (metabolism) and to reduce cholesterol and triglyceride levels. The mice were also rendered insulin resistant before the trial and started the trial obese. A high butyrate diet increased their insulin resistance and reduced their body weight.

Note: Besides taking your prebiotic fiber every day, butter is the best dietary source of butyrate, which got its name from butter.

Probiotics

These are designed to deliver live beneficial bacteria to the gut. I suggest that you consider making yourself fermented foods that deliver living probiotics in much higher doses. Homemade fermented foods are a staple of just about every known culture and besides tasting a whole lot better than a store-bought pill, they also cost a lot less.

If you want to buy your probiotics, you will find a profusion of different kinds available on the market. I suggest you try some different brands over a period of time; hopefully while you develop the (meager) skills required to make your own fermented foods.

One of the reasons that there are so many different kinds of commercial probiotics is that packaging a probiotic formulation that actually delivers live bacteria after being shipped and then standing on a store shelf at various temperatures, represents quite a challenge.

Besides the logistical challenges, any live bacteria that actually make it into the mouth of a consumer still have to survive the passage through the acid bath in the stomach.

Here are some of the probiotic bacteria you should find in good supplements:

Lactobacilli listed below have proven scientific value.[66] Some of them may also be effective against bladder infections.
- Acidophilus
- Reuteri
- Rhamnosus
- Casei
- Fermentum

Bifidobacteria make up about 25% of bacteria found in the colons of adults. The animalis variety is found in high levels in fermented dairy products and has been shown to survive gastric transit.[67]
- Bifidum
- Longum
- Animalis

Postbiotics

These kinds of substances are produced by the bacteria themselves and are not normally taken by mouth. There have been some attempts to create oral postbiotics using heat-killed bacteria. This method delivers the beneficial substances, which include butyrate, without the possible danger of administering live bacteria.[68]

Practically speaking, at the moment you cannot take a postbiotic, but you can ensure the promotion of their growth in your gut by taking pre- and probiotics and ensuring that you stay away from sugar and junk food.

Joint pain from your gut

As you have read elsewhere in this book, leaky gut and an abnormal gut microbiome affects your joints. I first discovered this in an unusual way. I found that my joint pain disappeared after suffering from a bout of explosive diarrhea. For a few days afterward, I felt on top of the world and ran around like a teenager.

The same thing happened to me on a few other occasions but at that time I had no idea why. I just knew that the 'runs' temporarily wrought a change in my gut, which made my arthritic psoriasis better.

Today, I have a better understanding of why this happened. I think that the expedited digestive flow I experienced flushed out some of the 'bad' bacteria. This reduced the toxins and the leakiness in my gut wall and almost immediately reduced the severity of my symptoms. Today, my gut environment has normalized and I have no more joint pain at all.

Somehow, by fixing my gut, the inflammation in my joints subsided.

I sincerely hope that once you have normalized your gut functions, by following the advice in this book, your joint pain will disappear too.

Milk: A2 vs. A1

There is range of dairy products produced that market the fact that they contain A2 protein. Scientists believe that a gene mutation in Holstein cows a few hundred years ago changed the structure of casein, the main protein in milk. They found that the milk of some cows contained the A2 variety of beta-casein, while others contained the A1 type.

African and Asian cows produce A2 milk, while European, American, Australian and New Zealand cows produce both A2 and A1.

The difference between A2 and A1 casein is small – just one amino acid difference. In A1 milk this amino acid is a histadine instead of a proline. To keep it simple, prolines have a rigid structure and are chemically slow to react. Histadines are much more reactive.

The presence of the histadine in the casein molecule causes a structural weakness in the casein. This weakness manifests during digestion when the molecule breaks into two parts at this weak link. One of the fragments produced is a seven-chain molecule called beta-casomorphin-7.

If you look at the end of that long name, you will be able to discern a word similar to morphine. Beta-casomorphin is categorized as an opioid, with some narcotic properties. It also seems to cause digestive problems in some people and is also possibly involved in heart disease, Type 1 diabetes, autism and schizophrenia.

Studies have shown that pepsin (an enzyme found in the gut) splits A1 milk in significant amounts and produces up to seven times more beta-casomorphin than is produced from A2 milk.[69]

Lastly, a study has questioned a possible link between Sudden Infant Death Syndrome (SIDS) and A1 milk producing high levels of beta-casomorphin. This is because of A1 milk's opioid properties, which may depress the respiratory center of some infants in a way similar to morphine.

Commerce

The A2 Corporation is a New Zealand company that produces the genetic test for A1 cows as well as methods of producing A2 herds. In some countries, like Australia, the sale of A2 milk provides a unique selling point for these brands of dairy products.

Recommendations

Although the jury is still out on the actual health consequences of consuming A1 milk[70], this has not stopped vocal support from many health professionals for A2 milk and the growth of A2-related commercial ventures.

I believe that there is probably some basis to the A1/A2 controversy, mainly because of studies that show higher opioid levels being produced from A1 milk. If you don't live in Africa or Asia and you are presented with the option of buying A2 milk, I suggest that you always opt for that variety.

While you are welcome to consume some dairy in fermented forms such as yogurt and kefir, butter and a little cream, **never drink milk of either variety**. The more fermented the dairy is, the fewer gut issues it will cause.

FODMAP

FODMAPs are carbohydrates (sugars) that are found in foods. The term FODMAP arises from attempts to treat patients with IBS (Irritable Bowel Syndrome). IBS covers a spectrum of gastrointestinal symptoms including: cramps, bloating, burping, excessive gas and diarrhea. It was proposed that foods containing fermentable carbohydrates, oligosaccharides (like fructans), disaccharides (like lactose), monosaccharides (like fructose) and polyols (like xylitol) were principally involved in causing many of the symptoms of IBS.

FODMAP-containing foods are poorly digested, especially when eaten in quantity. They are fermented by the gut bacteria, producing gas in the process, which leads to pressure in the gut. This pressure then causes most of the symptoms of IBS.

DIET: THE FIRST HORSEMAN

Many people with FODMAP sensitivity automatically avoid some food with FODMAPs because they have disagreed with them in the past.

The diet in this book restricts many of the FODMAP-containing foods. However, it does include dairy in the form of cream, yoghurt or butter. If you have a history of IBS or suffer from some of the IBS symptoms, I suggest that you exclude dairy from your diet, especially in the first few months. Fruit contains high FODMAP levels, but as this diet restricts most fruit except berries, you should be OK.

The other important area to watch out for is vegetables. Many veggies have high FODMAP levels, so be careful of eating large portions of them. I have listed some below, but if you have IBS, it is better to avoid any but the smallest portion of veggies during the first few months.

Veggies containing FODMAPs

- Asparagus
- Artichoke
- Beetroot
- Brinjal (eggplant)
- Broccoli
- Brussels sprouts
- Butternut
- Cabbage
- Celery
- Cauliflower
- Corn (sweet corn)
- Fennel
- Garlic
- Leek
- Mushrooms
- Onion
- Radish
- Sweet potato
- Squash

Cereal grains

Cereals are grasses that produce edible grain. In modern societies, cereal grains provide by far the greatest portion of available food.

Grains have only recently been domesticated by man for use as food. By recently, I mean in the last 10,000 years or less. In evolutionary terms, 10,000 years is the blink of an eye. Man has been evolving for a few million years and men and women like us have been around almost unchanged for over 100,000 years.

This recent domestication of wild grasses has exposed humans to many new species of antigens and produced a wide array of new challenges to our immune systems. Genetic manipulation of wheat has produced the now dominant dwarf wheat grown worldwide. The genetic changes in dwarf wheat expose us to many new antigens and proteins.

Cereal production

Maize (corn), wheat and rice account for about 90% of world cereal production.[71] Other grasses produced include:
- Barley
- Sorghum
- Millet
- Oats
- Rye
- Triticale
- Buckwheat
- Quinoa

The worst mistake

A famous essay by Jared Diamond published in 1987 argued that agriculture bequeathed a catastrophe on mankind. Rather than being the facilitator that allowed us to create large stable societies, Diamond sees agriculture as the cause of social and sexual inequalities as well as the rampant disease and despotism that plague modern life.[72]

Irrespective of the social challenges that agriculture brought upon us, the health challenges are just as severe and much closer to us on an individual level.

Many experts agree that some people's bodies struggle to defend them against the grains that are in our food supply. If you have an autoimmune disease, you are probably one of them.

Bisphenol A (BPA)

Bisphenol A (BPA) is used in the production of many plastic articles such as water and baby bottles, thermal printouts for till slips and parking tickets. BPA is also used in the manufacture of plastic films like food wraps, polystyrene items and take-away coffee cups.

Bisphenol A interferes with the production, secretion, transport, action, function and elimination of natural hormones. BPA can imitate our hormones in a way that can be hazardous to our health. Babies and young children are said to be especially sensitive to the effects of BPA.

Thermal printouts

Many thermal printers, like those that produce till slips, ATM receipts and parking tickets, use BPA as part of the inking process.

A simple rule with thermal printouts: regard all of them as potentially dangerous.

- Never put one in your mouth as I see so many people do when they pay for parking and need a free hand to search for change.
- Never handle one of these slips when you have hand cream or grease on your hands; the oils dramatically increase the concentration of BPA that leaches out of the print into your skin.

Plastic food containers

- Don't store food in plastic containers unless you have no choice (use glass whenever possible).

- Don't use plastic water bottles to carry water around.
- Store bottled water in glass bottles whenever possible.
- Never reuse a plastic bottled water bottle – it is made of the cheapest and least durable plastic possible and is intended for a single use only.
- Never microwave or heat food in plastic containers.
- Don't wash plastic containers in strong detergents or with hot water.

Good phytate, bad phytate

Plants store phosphorus as phytate (or phytic acid). The highest concentrations of phytates are found in grains, nuts and seeds. Humans cannot digest phytates, unlike cows and sheep. Phytates have mixed effects on the gut; they are less beneficial in the small intestine and more beneficial in the large intestine.

Since humans have been exposed to phytates for hundreds of thousands of years, I am confident that we need some phytates in our diet. That said, we probably don't need too much either. Levels of phytates are highest in seeds with sesame seed being the highest. As for nuts, Brazil nuts and almonds have the highest levels, with hazelnuts having the lowest.[73]

Effect on minerals

It is well known that high levels of phytates reduce absorption of minerals in the small intestine. The minerals mostly affected are iron and zinc. During absorption, the phytic acid binds to these minerals, making them unavailable for absorption. Vegans have a diet high in phytates and as a result are prone to anemia.

Benefits

It has been suggested that phytates have anti-cancer and cardio-protective properties. Some studies have demonstrated tumor growth inhibition by phytates and the lower levels of iron they cause may reduce colon cancer rates. While in the cardiovascular system, phytates may reduce plaque formation in artery walls as well as having an effect on platelets.

Issues

Some of the problems that high phytate consumption may cause are:
- Reduced absorption of iron and minerals
- Constipation
- Reduced digestion of fats and proteins because of interaction with digestive enzymes

Soaking and heating nuts

You can reduce phytate levels by soaking or heating your nuts before you eat them. This is similar to the way in which we treat beans to make them digestible.

Take home message on phytates

We do need some phytates in our food supply, just not too much. Eating nuts (as proposed in the Diet section of this program), will increase your phytate consumption. Be aware of that and do not 'pig out' on nuts. Simply limit your consumption to a handful of nuts on some days. Also be on the lookout for the constipation that excess nut consumption may cause.

Why you shouldn't use sweeteners

Logically, it makes no sense to substitute sugar, a known health hazard, with other substances whose health risks are unknown. Irrespective of any risks, the worldwide sweetener marketing machine manages to achieve sales of over 30 million tons of the stuff annually.[74] So much for being logical! What's more, the sales of sugar substitutes are growing faster than the sales of sugar and high fructose corn syrup.[75]

So many of my patients sit calmly when I tell them to abandon bread and sweet fruits, but get wide-eyed and indignant when I tell them to stop using sweeteners. 'They have no calories, Doc!' is the normal opening argument, but calorie content is not actually the issue, and I reply, 'These things are so smart that they make you fatter without the calories.'

Fatter

Sweeteners make you fat in two major ways.

First, sweeteners stimulate appetite and thus drive consumption of additional calories. This finding is supported by a number of large, credible studies. A 2010 Yale review found that sweeteners don't activate the normal food-reward pathways in the brain in the same way that sugar does and so the brain does not register sweeteners as having a satiating effect[76]. This can lead to increased food intake.

In the second place, sweeteners raise the level of insulin and leptin. Higher blood insulin enhances fat storage, which soon results in increased hunger. The leptin regulates body weight, food intake, as well as the body's use of energy. Prolonged high leptin levels are profoundly bad for your health and besides promoting obesity, can affect cognitive functions as well as brain energy metabolism.[77]

My biggest issue with swapping sugar for sweeteners is that they maintain 'the taste of sweet'. Rather than finding a means to control sugar urges, sweeteners perpetuate the urge to eat sweet things.

Gut bugs

Somehow, the bugs in our gut seem to be tied into our body-weight. It now appears that artificial sweeteners also have an effect on our gut bacteria. Chemicals in the sweeteners seem to alter the ratio of the two dominant groups of gut bacteria, Bacteroides and Firmicutes. In tests, this change in bacterial composition produced insulin resistance in the test mice. It took just 11 weeks for normal FDA approved doses of aspartame, sucralose or saccharin to produce glucose intolerance and dysbiosis in the test mice.[78]

The message is clear: if you want to fix your gut, you have to stop consuming all forms of artificial sweeteners.

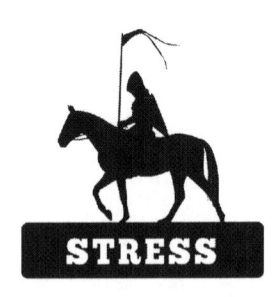

STRESS: The Second Horseman

The fact that stress affects our gut in terms of leakiness and absorptive ability is well known. What is not so well known is that stress affects the composition of the bacterial colonies in our gut. As I mentioned earlier, a study of Russian pilots found that the stress of combat could totally wipe out a pilot's bug population.

Newer studies have demonstrated similar results. A 2011 study of mice showed an immediate change in their gut bacteria in response to socially disruptive stress. Particular populations of colon bacteria were affected, significantly a reduction in the population size of the genus Bacteroides. The 'holes' left by these bacteria were filled by members of the Firmicutes genus Clostridii.

Having more Firmicutes than Bacteroides sounds like gobbledygook, but it has implications in our diet that are the focus of much research. There appears to be a close relationship between body weight and how many Bacteroides you have in your gut. More Bacteroides, less body fat. To me, this makes it clear that this is one important way that stress makes you fat.

I am confident that there will be more and more studies linking stress to biome changes as interest in this field of study grows.

Cortisol

Cortisol is your stress hormone. It is produced in the adrenal glands, which are small nut-sized organs that ride more or less on the top of the kidneys. The adrenals squirt cortisol into the bloodstream in response to stressful events.

Cortisol plays an important role in nutrition and it works through several mechanisms to increase blood sugar levels. In extreme circumstances, cortisol can also increase fat and protein breakdown. Certain immune functions are also suppressed, specifically in the area of inflammatory responses.

Normally, our cortisol levels fluctuate over the course of the day, peaking soon after we wake up and reaching its lowest level in the early hours of the morning.

We are mainly concerned with persistently high cortisol levels, caused mostly by stress.

The old fight or flight response gone crazy

In a stress situation, a quick burst of adrenaline, mixed with some cortisol, is just the ticket for a 'flight or fight' response. However, when cortisol levels remain high, as they do in chronic stress, then bad things happen.

High blood levels of cortisol can:
- Create sugar cravings
- Increase water retention

- Affect digestion
- Increase fat storage tendencies
- Raise your blood pressure
- Disturb sleeping patterns
- Drop testosterone levels in males
- Disrupt menstrual cycles in women
- Delay healing
- Weaken bones

Adrenal fatigue

This is the stage where, after a long period of producing high levels of cortisol in response to chronic stress, the adrenal glands become unable to produce sufficient levels to support normal daily bodily functions. Because it is a difficult diagnosis to make conclusively, some medical professionals do not credit it as a real illness.

> **'... it's safe to assume that adrenal fatigue is the most prevalent fake disease in the world.'**[79]

People suffering from this condition often have mild depression accompanied by extreme tiredness, often in the mid-afternoon. They may also experience sleep disturbances and weight gain.

Either way, real or unreal, symptoms of adrenal fatigue or chronic stress trouble many people and lowering stress levels will certainly help them to feel better.

Note: Cortisone is not the same thing as cortisol, although they have similar actions. When used as a medicine, cortisol is called hydrocortisone.

Oxytocin: The hugging hormone

Oxytocin is a hormone produced in an area of the brain called the hypothalamus. It has long been known to play a pivotal role in childbirth, where it works on the uterus during labor. After birth, it is produced during breast feeding, creating sensations that enhance mother-child bonding.

More recently, oxytocin has been found to be released in both sexes by a range of activities. These include:

- Sexual activities
- Social activities
- Person to person behavior

Oxytocin produces calming sensations and reduces anxiety. It has also been suggested that oxytocin is released to enhance feelings of trust and belonging in group situations.

Stress buster

Paul Zak (Dr Love) is famous for his recommendation that hugging or being hugged at least eight times a day leads to a more enjoyable life, with improved relationships.

Our main interest in oxytocin is its ability to reduce stress by lowering cortisol levels. You can use your knowledge of how to stimulate oxytocin's release to increase your feel-better state emotionally and to lower your cortisol levels. Doing these kinds of activities on a daily basis will have a profoundly beneficial effect on your health.

Keep on:
- Hugging the people around you who you care about
- Touching people when possible and when permissible

- Being intimate with your mate by doing things like holding hands and touching
- Having sex as often as possible

Oxytocin in medical therapy

Although it has been investigated for use in a number of conditions, at this stage oxytocin supplementation is by no means a standard therapy for any condition. It has been tested as a therapy for post-partum depression, Post-Traumatic Stress Disorder (PTSD) and in a small study of schizophrenia. Another study found that it normalized brain activity responsible for social behaviors in children with autism (ASD).[80]

Automatic nervous system

Actually called the Autonomic Nervous System (ANS), it controls our automatic (involuntary) body functions such as digestion, breathing, sweating, heartbeat and blood pressure. In other words, the ANS controls parts of our bodies without any conscious effort on our part.

The organs the ANS controls include:

- Stomach
- Digestive glands
- Lungs
- Heart
- Intestines
- Kidneys
- Bladder
- Pupils

The ANS is divided into two parts: Sympathetic and Parasympathetic. These two parts of the ANS work together to ensure that the automatic functions of our bodies adjust to suit our environment and our physical requirements.

In general, the sympathetic system controls organs in stressful situations and is the 'fight or flight' part of the ANS. In modern terms it is also called the 'quick response system'.

The parasympathetic system is involved in restful situations and helps the body to recover and rest. It is the 'rest and digest' or 'feed and breed' part of the ANS.

One way to visualize how the activities of these two systems counterbalance each other is to view them as:

- Sympathetic – Speeds up, increases alertness and tension
- Parasympathetic – Relaxes and calms, lowers blood pressure, increases digestion

Most organs are connected to both of these systems and operate based on a balance between their two inputs. It works almost like the accelerator and the foot brake in a car. In daily life, most of us run around in sympathetic nervous dominance, which means we tend towards 'fight or flight'. This means our 'rest and digest' functions take a back seat.

One of the goals of this book is to teach you ways to promote control of your parasympathetic system at certain times of the day. We normally use breath control, which you can read more about in the Breathing Control section in Stress to drive this.

Physical signs of sympathetic dominance

There are some signs you can look for, which will help you gauge your physical state of sympathetic stimulation.

How tense your jaw and neck muscles are, is a good place to start. You know that moment when you realize that your jaw is so tightly clenched that if you don't relax a little, you're going to need the Jaws of Life to open it. Poor balance or clumsiness is another sign of tense muscles. Your breathing is another dead giveaway. Rapid shallow breaths are a sure sign that your ANS is out of balance.

It has sexual effects too. Males suffer from premature ejaculation and females from an inability to orgasm because their pelvic muscles are too tightly wound.

Constipation is another effect of sympathetic over-stimulation..

Mental signs of sympathetic dominance

These are easy to spot but become so much a part of us that we don't even realize it.
- Sense of urgency
- Inability to relax
- Racing thoughts
- Impatience
- Controlling behavior
- Outbursts of anger

Heart rate variability (HRV)

Measuring the variability of the time interval between heartbeats is a technique that is in wide use. It has seen extensive use in research and medical diagnostics, being used to predict higher mortality risk in heart attack victims, depression and survival rates in premature babies, to name but a few examples. Athletes use HRV to measure the effects of training and can extend rest periods between activities when their HRV shows that they need more recovery time.

There are programs available that target HRV as a means of measuring and reducing sympathetic over-stimulation. One of these is from The Heart Math Institute. Their Inner Balance Program connects your heart rhythms to your iPhone by means of a small earlobe connector. The program shows you how to achieve 'coherence, which is state of synchronization between your heart, brain and autonomic nervous system'.

The bottom line

Your parasympathetic nervous system needs constant attention. Left to its own devices, it soon slips back into being submissive to the demands of 'fight or flight' dominance.

Work on it consciously. Insist on your daily dose of quiet-time and be as mindful of your breathing as you can, especially in stressful situations or environments. Keep working at being positive. Relax those muscles, your stiff jaw and tense neck. Smile at yourself in the mirror.

ACTIVITY: The Third Horseman

Exercise variations

Here are some of the ways in which you can change and vary your activities. Variations will keep you from getting bored and can also be used to alter intensity levels.

The exercise variations below can be applied to any exercise you do. On occasion, they can also be used back-to-back in a single session.

Interval training

Interval training is suitable for any level of activity. It is used to train Olympic athletes and is just as applicable to you. An interval session is a short session.

An interval workout alternates bouts of high intensity work with lower intensity work, or sometimes rest. You can change your interval workouts by increasing high intensity periods and reducing rest periods, or vice versa.

Here is an example of how interval training can be used for walking or running:

- Warm up for 10 minutes
- Walk or jog for 60 seconds
- Sprint or walk as fast as you can for 30 seconds
- Rest for 60 seconds
- Repeat five or 10 times

As you can see from the example above, it is easy to change the interval routine. Just by lengthening the sprint phase or removing it, you can completely change the exercise.

Here is another, simpler interval variation.

- Warm up for 10 minutes
- Increase your pace at regular intervals until you are at maximum effort
- Slow the pace to walking or jogging for as long as it takes you to recover completely
- Repeat

Intervals are tiring so don't do them on consecutive days. Always have a rest day after an interval session.

Long slow climb

This variation effectively makes a hill when there isn't one available. It works by gradually increasing load as you do the workout, as if you are climbing a hill that gets steadily steeper. It can be done on many types of equipment.

On a treadmill: Warm up at a comfortable pace for up to 10 minutes and then increase either the speed or the incline (or both) at regular intervals. Stop when you can go no more.

Russian steps

This type of training varies the pace at set time intervals, building to a crescendo and then slowing back down at set intervals. You can imagine it as a series of steady climbs up to a peak and then a steady climb down.

Here is a difficult version used by Roger Iddles, a cycling World Masters Champion, which is based on 10-minute intervals (which you can shorten if you like).

- Warm up for 10 minutes
- Ride, walk, jog, etc. as hard as you can for one minute
- Rest by going slowly for nine minutes
- Add another minute to the hard as you can go interval
- Reduce the rest period by one minute
- Repeat until you are going as hard as you can for nine minutes with a one minute rest
- To come down, decrease the hard interval in one minute intervals and increase rest intervals by the same amount

Russian steps are hard, so never do more than one session of these per week.

Myokines

We are just beginning to understand the complicated signaling network that our organs use to communicate with one another. Signals are sent between cells using small protein molecules, collectively called cytokines. Cytokines affect the behavior of the target cells and sometimes themselves. They are sometimes classified according to the cell type they originate from; adipokines come from fat cells (adipocytes), interleukins are from white blood cells (leucocytes), and myokines are released from muscle cells.

We are interested in skeletal muscle myokines which, when released from muscle cells, affect a wide range of body functions, some of which include regeneration, repair and immunity. They also act on the muscles themselves.

It appears that each bout of exercise produces a generalized anti-inflammatory effect, which provides a defense against chronic diseases. This is another good reason to exercise regularly.[81]

Largest organ

If we look at skeletal muscle as a single entity, it constitutes the largest organ in the body. When muscles contract they release chemicals that affect other organs in the body, and as they are collectively such a large organ, activities that engage many muscles can potentially have a major effect on the rest of the body.

Contracting muscles release myokines, which contribute to metabolic changes as well as to adaptations to the activity load. Some of these changes are anti-inflammatory and provide protection against chronic inflammatory diseases such as insulin resistance and hardening of the arteries. Muscle contraction causes the release of a cascade of myokines[82], which include:
- Irisin (increases breakdown of stored fat)
- IL-15 (increases muscle mass)
- LIF (aids muscle regeneration)
- BDNF (oxidizes fat)
- FGF-21 (increases glucose uptake)
- SPARC (down-regulates fat storage in adipocytes)

Myokines released during activity also exert an effect on fat tissue by speeding up fat release and antagonizing fat cell adipokines. The muscles themselves are also affected by myokines released during activity and enhance glucose transport as well as fat breakdown.

Diabetes

Much of the research on myokines has been in the area of diabetes and the metabolic syndrome. Most of this research points to the positive effects of myokine release during and after exercise, the effects of which are:
- Lowered average blood glucose levels
- Reduction in systemic inflammation markers
- Decreased cardiac risk factors
- Reduced body mass
- Reduced diabetes medication requirements

SLEEP: The Fourth Horseman

Your sleep clock

What we are really trying to do when we work on your sleep patterns is to normalize your internal clock. In medical terms, this is called your circadian rhythm, which exists in all living creatures and runs in 24-hour cycles. The term circadian is derived from Latin and loosely means 'around the day'.

Circadian clocks are driven internally but also listen to outside signals, especially light. The rhythm of these clocks allow for sleeping periods of rest, followed by waking hours of work.

In humans 'the clock' is a cluster of cells in the brain in an area called the hypothalamus. These cells are wired to the retina in the eye and react to light entering the eye. This is the primary reason why dimming your environment at night is so important for your sleep.

Humans living without electricity have circadian clocks that directly follow periods of day and night. Unfortunately, our modern environment disrupts these rhythms.

Hopefully, you can use the methods outlined in the sleep section to reset your body clock so that you can sleep better and heal your body.

Opposite is a diagram representing a circadian rhythm of a fictional person who goes to sleep at about 10pm and wakes at around 6am. It will give you an idea of how your circadian rhythm works and how different body processes are affected by the time of day.

The detail for the timing of the various body events was taken from a book about the use of circadian rhythm timing to optimize treatment times (Chronotherapy).[84] The authors propose that the timing of therapies for chronic diseases is an important factor in the healing process.

This is yet another indication of how important regulating your body clock is to achieving the best possible health.

SLEEP: THE FOURTH HORSEMAN

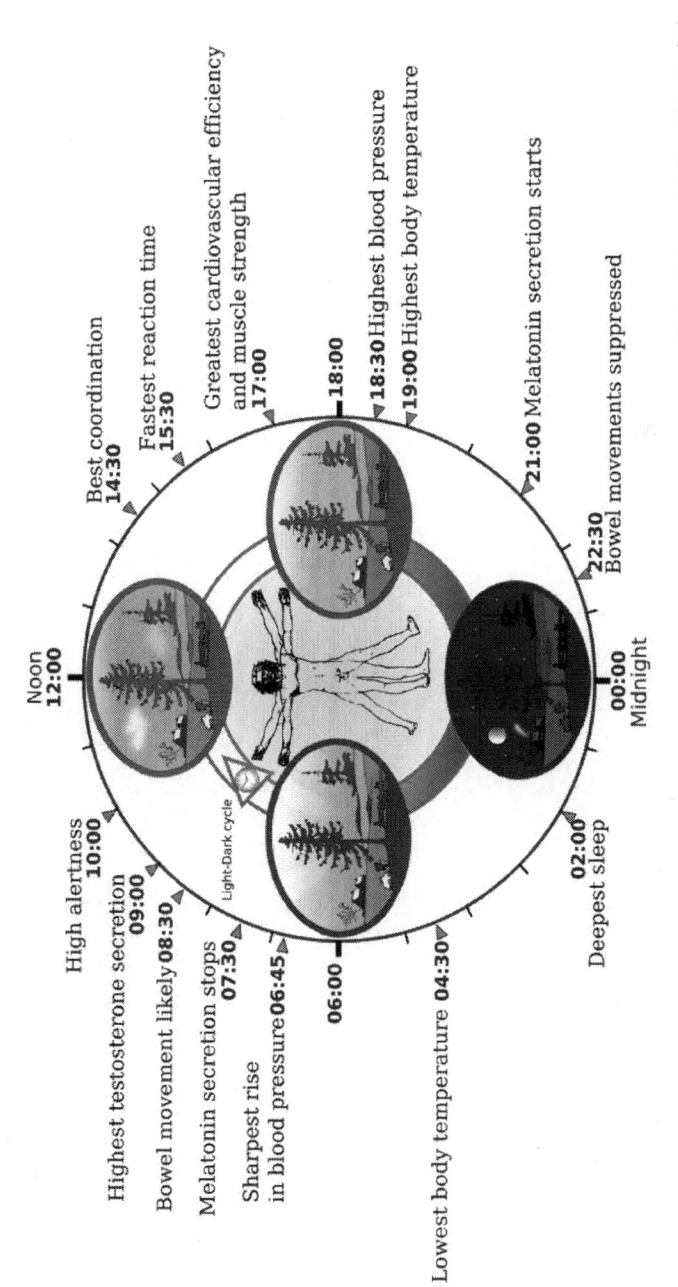

RESOURCES

Recipes

Gut healing recipes

If you are looking for recipes suitable for this diet, there are many good sources. Look for low-carb or LCHF recipes; most of these will be good for your diet because they replace sugars with fat.

I have however provided some special gut healing recipes and would go so far as to say that you have to use at least one or two of these every week.

The recipes explained

- The two soups are great gut-healers and immune support foods
- The chocolate coconut treats are a tasty way to get butter into your daily diet. You don't have to make them every day but you do have to make sure you eat some butter every day!
- The fermented food recipes are starter guides to get you going along the route to eating something fermented every day. These foods are super foods in terms of prebiotics, vitamins and minerals. Once you get started, I am sure that you will start to feel so much better that you will want to explore the world of fermented foods. A friendly place to start is at Donna Schwenk's Cultured Food Life (culturedfoodlife.com).

Let's begin with two bone broth recipes!

Gail's bone marrow soup

Ingredients:
- 4–6 fresh marrow bones (not defrosted)
- 2–3 medium-sized fresh pieces of soup meat (not defrosted)
- 3 medium carrots, sliced
- 3 sticks of celery broken up (no leaves)
- 2 leeks, finely sliced (or an onion if you don't have leeks)
- 2 chopped turnips
- 3 medium slices of pumpkin
- 1–2 cubes of your favorite chicken stock
- Don't forget to add some flavoring using herbs you enjoy; also add some natural salt and pepper.

Method:
- Bring the bones and meat to a boil and simmer for one hour (skim off the scum from the water regularly).
- In a deep soup pot lightly sauté the veggies in butter or olive oil, together with the flavoring. Then add the cooked bones and meat and stock. Cover with water and cook for three hours on medium to low heat until the meat is soft.

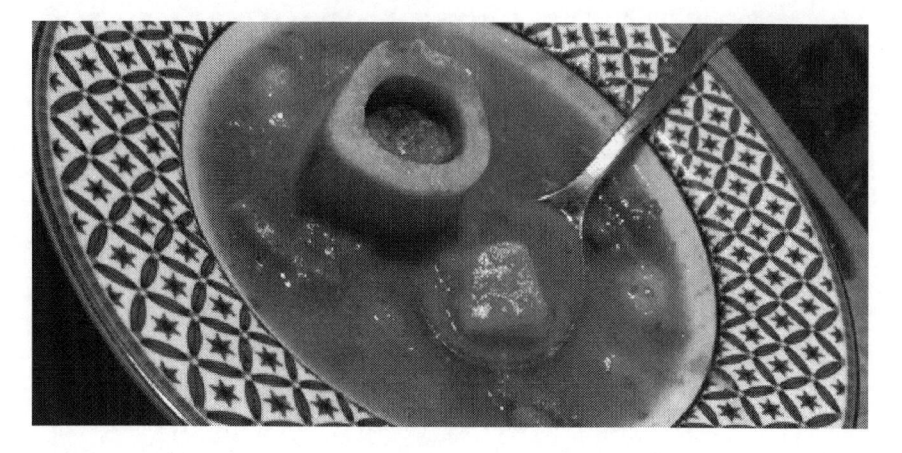

Gail's whole chicken soup

Ingredients:
- I medium-large fresh chicken (organic if possible and not defrosted)
- 2 medium carrots
- 4–5 sticks of celery broken up (keep leaves separate)
- 1 onion quartered
- ½ butternut
- 3 medium slices of pumpkin
- 1 chicken stock cube or alternately use a good chicken stock
- Flavoring: your favorite herbs and seasonings with some coarse natural salt and pepper, and paprika. Add a sprinkling of chili flakes if you like a kick (avoid during Detox and use sparingly during Maintenance).

Method:
- Place the chicken in a deep pot with all the veggies. Cover with water, add flavoring (including the chicken stock) and bring to a slow boil.
- Allow the chicken and veggies to simmer for at least 2–3 hours (or longer), until the chicken falls off the bone.
- You can add additional water and stock if you're left with mostly chicken.

Refrigerate any leftovers and reheat when you are ready for more. It seems to taste better and better the longer it lasts!

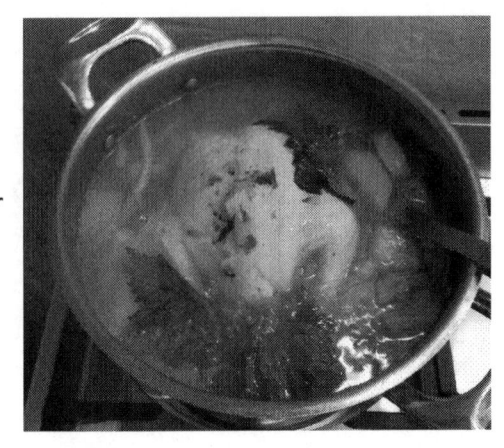

Paige's chocolate coconut treats

These are so good for your gut that they should be called medicine balls. They are also easy to make and store in the fridge for a daily treat.

The key ingredient is butter, which tastes as good to us as it does to our gut lining. The butyrate in butter has evolved to be a primary source of energy for the cells lining our gut. The butyrate heals the gut lining and decreases permeability (makes it less leaky).

Ingredients:
- 2 cups of dessicated coconut
- 3 tablespoons of melted coconut oil
- 4 tablespoons of melted butter
- 1 tablespoon of cocoa powder
- 1 teaspoon of vanilla essence

Method:
- Blend the ingredients together
- Roll into balls or spoon into a muffin tin
- Allow to set in the refrigerator for 20 minutes
- Store in a container in the refrigerator

Homemade sauerkraut

This is the easiest fermented food you can make. There are many variations you can use to extend my basic sauerkraut recipe below.

Sauerkraut contains many live bacteria (mainly lactobacilli).[90] Eating sauerkraut, is a much more practical and tasty way of loading good bacteria into your gut, than buying probiotics.

Ingredients:
- 1 whole cabbage (preferably organically grown). You can use more than one, or even mix different color cabbages.
- Natural salt like Himalayan (don't use white commercial salt if you can help it)

Optional ingredients: A few slices of horseradish to add taste and prevent mold from forming.

You will also need a sharp knife or a slicer to chop the cabbage, and a crock to ferment the cabbage in. There are proper commercial crocks available, but a strong glass jar will do for smaller quantities.

To cover your jar, you can use the original stopper that came with it – closed lightly but not tightly. Alternatively, you can cover your jar with a fine-weave cloth, which must remain damp to limit the entry of air. Oxygen is not your friend here; too much exposure to air will cause your sauerkraut to create vinegar (acetic acid) and ruin it.

Method:
- Chop the cabbage into thin slices using the knife or a slicer
- Mix some salt into the sliced cabbage (don't make it too salty)
- Leave your cabbage and salt mixture overnight, if you have the time. It softens the cabbage and draws the water out.
- If you are using the horseradish, drop a few pieces into the bottom of your fermentation container. (Go easy on the quantity of horseradish you use; it has quite a strong kick!)
- Then fill your fermentation jar with sliced cabbage.
- If you are using the horseradish, you can add a few more pieces halfway through.
- The jar must be two thirds full; never fill to the brim.
- Now you need to crush the cabbage as hard as you can. Most people use their hands or fists. Some German purists crush it with their feet, or you can use a wooden plunger to do it.

- You know you're crushing it properly when water starts to form.
- If there is not enough water to cover the top of the cabbage in the fermentation jar, add some filtered water until the cabbage is underwater.
- Place a weight on top of the cabbage to keep it below water level. I use a glass bottle, but you can use any clean glass or porcelain object. If you use stones make sure they have been properly sterilized!
- Cover the jar. (If you seal it, be sure to open it every day because fermentation makes gas that can cause the jar to explode.)

Daily maintenance:

Depending on the temperature it is stored at, the sauerkraut will need anything between one to three weeks to ferment.

You must check it every day:

- Push the cabbage below the waterline, making sure that you push hard and long enough to release any bubbles trapped in the cabbage
- Smell it carefully; it should have a strong smell but must never have a bad smell.
- It should not turn a brown color.
- The film on top of the water should never be of a creamy consistency.

By day five or day seven, you can start tasting your sauerkraut. Keep doing this until you find the taste that suits you, then decant and refrigerate. Your sauerkraut is ready for eating!

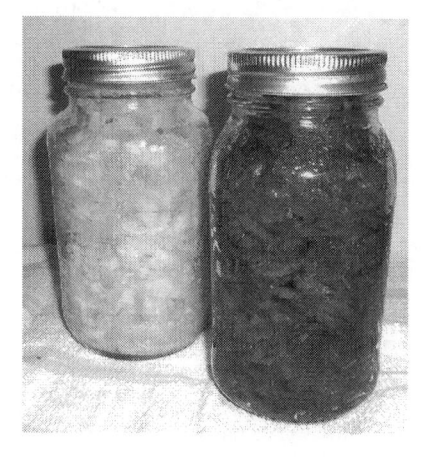

Watch for mold formation – it is not desirable. It will form at the top of the water or on the topmost layer of the cabbage. If this happens to you, you can try to skim it off along with the top layer of cabbage. This should stop any more mold from forming. If it does not, throw everything out and sterilize the bottle and any equipment you used and start again.

Milk kefir

This is another super-easy fermented food to make. It tastes like drinking yogurt. Kefir is full of friendly lactobacilli, yeast and vitamins. There is no fixed content of beneficial nutrients because they will vary depending on the milk you use. Vitamins and minerals that will probably be in your kefir include: Vitamin B12 and K2 as well as the minerals calcium and magnesium.

Milk kefir will boost your immunity and help heal your gut. I make and drink it almost every day.

Your biggest challenge will be sourcing the kefir grains you will need to ferment the milk. The best way, I found, was to locate someone living near you who makes kefir. A quick Facebook search found a number of people in my area who had grains. Most people will be happy to give you some grains because one of the products of making kefir is more grains! There are also many internet stores that will send you some. Preferably obtain live grains instead of the frozen or freeze-dried types.

Ingredients:
- Two teaspoons of kefir grains
- Half a quart (500ml) of fresh cow's or goat's milk

Method:
- Pour the milk into a clean glass jar
- Add the kefir grains

- Cover the jar with a cloth or use a paper coffee filter secured with a rubber band
- Leave on a warm shelf

How long you let your kefir stand is up to you. A 24-hour cycle usually works well but it may take longer in cold climates. Taste some. If it still tastes like milk, you need to wait longer. If it gets tart too quickly, maybe you have used too many grains. Stop when the taste is right for you, but remember the longer it ferments, the better it is for you.

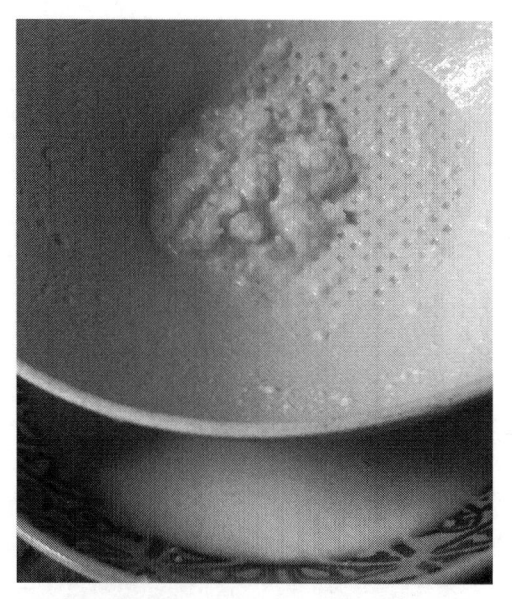

Do not be put off if your kefir separates into a creamy top part, with a clear liquid bottom. It can also develop into lumps that don't look that tasty. Relax. A quick stir with a wooden spoon will mix it all together into a nice milky consistency.

Decanting your kefir

You will need a fairly coarse strainer and a container. Simply place your strainer over the container and pour. The kefir grains will be caught by the strainer, as in the image below. You can refrigerate the kefir and put the grains into a new batch of milk.

Some tips: If you need to stop making kefir for a while, tightly seal your grains with some milk in a glass container and store in the refrigerator until you need them again. I have a permanent kefir storage container in my refrigerator.

The grain colonies used to activate fermentation will expand naturally. As the colonies grow larger they begin to ferment my milk too quickly. When this happens I pour them into the storage container, stir, and then take out a new batch to ferment with.

Slippery Elm tea

This is a simple, tasty tea you can prepare in minutes.

Ingredients:
- Slippery Elm powder
- Warm water

Method:
- Add a heaped teaspoon of Slippery Elm to a mug or coffee cup
- Fill the cup with some warm (not boiling) water
- Stir
- Leave for a few minutes and then stir again
- Drink

The stuff does not look that appetizing! But it tastes good.

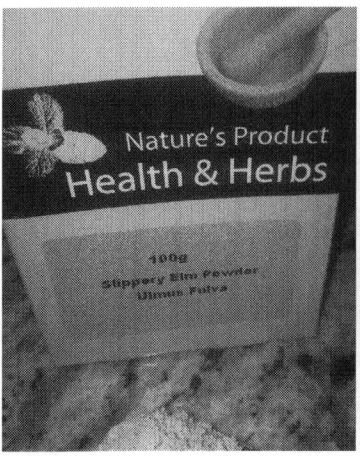

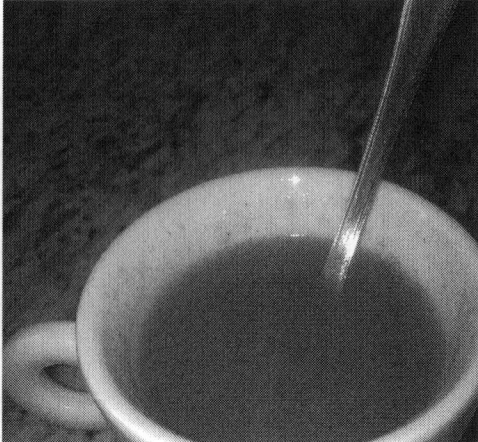

I drink a cup first thing in the morning on an empty stomach and wait for about 30 minutes before I take any supplements, drinks or food.

If you are taking any medications, the mucilage in Slippery Elm may possibly slow absorption, although there is no real evidence of this. As a precaution, wait an hour at least or even two hours before taking your meds, to be sure they will be absorbed.

Kombucha

Make yourself a tasty drink that is packed with good bacteria, yeast, vitamins and minerals.

Before you start, you will need a SCOBY. You can find one locally from someone who makes kombucha or else SCOBYs can be ordered from various Internet outlets. A SCOBY is a Symbiotic Colony of Bacteria and Yeast.

It does not look that appealing but the kombucha it makes is.

Ingredients:
- SCOBY
- 4 green tea bags (or you can try with any other herbal tea)
- Sugar (to feed the SCOBY, not you!)

You will need a large glass jar to hold your SCOBY and the tea.

Method:
- Boil sufficient filtered water in a pot to fill your glass jar two thirds
- Once the water has boiled, add the tea bags (turn the heat off)
- Add about four tablespoons of sugar
- Allow the tea to steep until it is cold
- Pour the cold tea into the glass jar (must be cold or it will kill your SCOBY)

- Drop your SCOBY into the tea
- Close the lid of the container loosely
- Store your jar somewhere warm in your kitchen

Now you need patience. It can take a week or two before things start to happen.

A new SCOBY will slowly form on the top of the tea. Once it starts becoming thick, you can taste the mixture. It will become less sweet as the SCOBYs eat the sugar. It is up to you to decide when to stop the process and pour out the kombucha, which will then be ready for drinking.

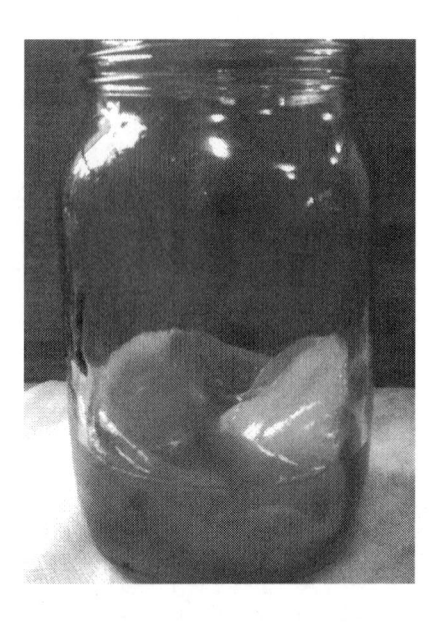

You will now have two SCOBYs, which is why people who brew kombucha are so happy to share them.

The key with kombucha is not to drink it sweet so as to avoid drinking too much sugar.

Second fermentation is another optional step in the process. After the SCOBY has been removed, you can add a small amount of sugar and a few pieces of some sweet fruit or vegetable, like ginger. When kept in a tightly-closed bottle for a few extra days, the added sugar will be fermented and will make the brew bubbly. It will also take on a new flavor if the source of the sugar was ginger, for example.

There are many Internet resources for kombucha fermentation that you can use to expand your kombucha-making abilities.

Guides

Green foods

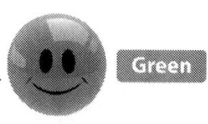

- Meat – eat the fatty bits if you can (lean meat on its own must be supplemented with fat)
- Any fish or seafood
- Poultry – chicken, turkey, duck (preferably free-range or organic)
- Veggies – eat lots of greens (see Vegetable Stoplight)
- Avocado (eat in abundance)
- Dairy – whole eggs (fry in butter, coconut oil or ghee)
- Dairy – butter, full cream yogurt
- Nuts – any except peanuts and cashews (watch your portion sizes!)
- Oils – olive oil, flax seed oil, coconut oil
- Mayonnaise – full fat (use sparingly)
- Water
- Chocolate – 85% or higher (not in excessive quantities)

Orange foods

These items can be eaten irregularly in small quantities. They should be tightly limited during Detox. They can be added during Maintenance but keep a careful check to see that you don't develop any signs of intolerance after eating them. Signs of intolerance include visible worsening of psoriasis plaques, stomach upsets, constipation and heart palpitations.

- Coffee (limited to 2 cups a day)
- Dairy – cream in the 2 cups of coffee a day, and some cheese is permissible

- Alcohol – limited to 1 double tot of non-grain spirit; a glass of dry white or dry red wine or sherry – three times a week
- Artificial sweeteners in the smallest possible quantities

Vegetables to eat in small portions

- Cabbage
- Eggplant (brinjals)
- Parsley
- Pumpkin
- Broccoli
- Turnips
- Fennel
- Kale
- Onions

Red foods

These foods are forbidden during Detox:
- Sugar (all colours)
- Honey, syrup or any honey substitute like (high fructose) corn syrup
- Bread of any kind including muffins, rolls, bagels
- Cereal grains – wheat, barley, maize, rye, sorghum, millet, buckwheat, quinoa and oats
- Any breakfast cereals – Wheaties, Post Toasties, Rice Krispies, oats, oat bran, etc.
- Milk (full fat cream can be used as a substitute) – do not use skim, 2% or low fat milk
- Fruit of any kind except berries
- Fruit juices of any kind
- Fructose in any form

- Yogurt, especially sweetened, low-fat or with fruit (only natural, Greek-type, double cream and non-sweetened high fat yogurt is allowed)
- Diet drinks
- Beer, fizzy alcoholic drinks, cocktails
- Starches of any kind (potatoes, rice, couscous, noodles, quinoa)
- Pasta of any kind including whole-wheat pasta
- Potatoes
- Margarines
- Vegetable oil except olive oil and flax seed oil
- All beans
- Carrots
- Peas
- Salad dressings that have sugar in them – stick to olive oil and a little balsamic if you are unsure (balsamic can be high in sugars)
- Ice-cream
- Sweets
- Sodas or sweetened drinks like Coke, lemonade, and so on
- Sports and energy drinks

Forbidden but not on the list

The above list of red items can never be complete. Sugar and refined carbs hide everywhere in your food supply so you will have to be eternally vigilant. If you start eating anything that tastes sweet – just stop; it is better to be safe than sorry.

Look out for hidden sugars. Many cooked items are made with sugar and other carbohydrate sweeteners, which 'they' forget to tell you about.

Some places you might find hidden danger:
- Sauces

- Salad dressings
- Cooked vegetables
- Fructose used as sweetener
- Honey hidden in a 'no-sugar added' treat

Always, always read the labels

Be wary of any store-bought food. Examine food labels for key words such as carbohydrates, glycemic sugars, glycemic 'anything', sugars and starch. Read and re-read the section "More on reading Nutrition Facts labels".

A study by the University of Carolina bought 85,451 uniquely formulated (branded) items from U.S. supermarkets between 2005 and 2009. They then tested each of these items for sugar content. An astounding 75% of these contained ADDED sugar, some of which were not discernible from the Nutrition Facts labeling.[91]

You are not alone: If you need advice or help with any item, please mail 4Horsemen@biohacks.guru and we will do our best to assist you.

Vegetable Stoplight

You must eat your veggies! But you need to be careful because some vegetables are high in carbs and are not suitable for eating during Detox.

You can eat:
- Freely from the green section
- Carefully from the orange section
- Sparingly from the red section

GUIDES

GREEN LIST	
Vegetable	Carbs/100g
Brussels sprouts	0.9
Watercress	1.3
Lettuces	2.0
Celery	3.0
Summer squash	3.1
Zucchini	3.1
Bean sprouts	3.2
Mushrooms	3.3
Endive	3.4
Radishes	3.4
Cucumber	3.6
Swiss chard	3.7
Asparagus	3.9
Spinach	3.9
Green beans	4.0
Tomatoes	4.0
Beet greens	4.3
Chives	4.4
Radicchio	4.5
Mustard greens	4.7
Cauliflower	5.0

ORANGE LIST	
Vegetable	Carbs/100g
Cabbage	5.8
Eggplant	5.9
Jalapeno peppers	5.9
Parsley	6.3
Pumpkin raw	6.5
Broccoli	6.6
Bell peppers	7.0
Snap beans	7.0
Turnip greens	7.1
Fennel	7.3
Kale	8.8
Dandelion greens	9.2
Onions	9.3

RED LIST	
Vegetable	Carbs/100g
Snap Peas	14.5
Shallots	16.8
Ginger Root	17.8
Hearts of Palm	25.6
Garlic	33.1

Parts from UMHS Adult Diabetes Education Program http://www.med.umich.edu/diabetes/education/ and from Diabetes.org.uk

Carbs in common nuts and seeds

Here is a list of carbohydrate counts in nuts:

Nut	Value per 100g
Brazil Nuts	12
Macadamia Nuts	14
Walnuts	14
Pecans	14
Peanuts	16
Hazelnuts	17
Almonds	22
Pistachios	28
Chestnuts	28
Cashews	30

Here is a list of carbohydrate counts in seeds. The chia seed rules; it is almost 50% carbohydrate.

Seed	Value per 100g
Pumpkin Seeds	11
Sunflower Seeds	20
Sesame Seeds	23
Flax Seeds	29
Chia Seeds	42

Charts

Bristol Stool Chart

If you need to know the answer to the question: 'What does normal poop look like?' then you have to ask someone who has looked at a lot of poop.

Luckily for us, Doctor Ken Heaton and some fellow doctors at the University of Bristol did just that. As a result, they were able to publish a chart of common poop shapes in 1997.

The doctors who did the research decided that there were seven basic stool (poop) shapes.[92] They published these as a reference chart that has, over the years, stood the test of time and is today regarded as reliable by medical authorities.[93],[94]

Note that the average person takes 24 to 72 hours to convert a meal to poop.

The ideal poop shape is Type 4 on the chart.

Poop types summary

Types 1 & 2 indicate some form of constipation

Types 3 & 4 are normal but Type 4 is preferred

Types 5, 6 & 7 indicate running stomach (diarrhea)

Type 1: Separate hard lumps, like nuts (hard to pass)
Poop of this shape and hardness indicate missing bacteria and a lack of in-transit fermentation. This kind of stool is sometimes seen in the

The Bristol Stool Chart

Type 1		Separate hard lumps, like nuts (hard to pass)
Type 2		Sausage-shaped but lumpy
Type 3		Like a sausage but with cracks on the surface
Type 4		Like a sausage or snake, smooth and soft
Type 5		Soft blobs with clear-cut edges
Type 6		Fluffy pieces with ragged edges, a mushy stool
Type 7		Watery, no solid pieces. Entirely Liquid

http://commons.wikimedia.org/wiki/File:Bristol_stool_chart.svg

Credits – Image of Bristol Chart:
Kyle Thompson derivative work: Jpb1301 [CC BY-SA 2.5-2.0-1.0 (http://creativecommons.org/licenses/by-sa/2.5-2.0-1.0), GFDL (www.gnu.org/copyleft/fdl.html) or CC-BY-SA-3.0 (http://creativecommons.org/licenses/by-sa/3.0/)], via Wikimedia Commons
License details: http://en.wikipedia.org/wiki/GNU_Free_Documentation_License

early stages of a low carb diet and can be fixed by the addition of more digestible fiber to the diet. Psyllium husks are a good choice for this.

Type 2: Sausage-shaped, but lumpy
This is a typical constipated poop, one that causes straining when it is passed. It is quite hard and dry, in a large sausage shape. Its dryness often indicates that it has spent significantly longer than normal in the colon. It can cause cracks in the anal ring (fissures) because it can be thicker than the anal outlet.

Type 3: Like a sausage but with cracks on its surface
Softer than the Type 2 sausage but still relatively hard to pass. They probably have a longer than normal bowel transit time.

Type 4: Like a sausage or snake, smooth and soft
The poop to aim for is a daily soft sausage, passed in long pieces.

Type 5: Soft blobs with clear-cut edges (passed easily)
Also a good poop. Sometimes similar to Type 4 but passed more than once a day.

Type 6: Fluffy pieces with ragged edges, a mushy stool
The poop is watery but still has some solid consistency. Too loose to be comfortable.

Type 7: Watery, no solid pieces, entirely liquid
Full-blown diarrhea with poop running like water.

Appendix

References

1. World Health Organization – Physical Activity.
   http://www.who.int/topics/physical_activity/en

2. Voigt, R.M., Forsyth, C.B., Green, S. J., Mutlu, E., Engen, P., Vitaterna, M. H., Turek, F. W., Keshavarzian A. (2014) Circadian Disorganization Alters Intestinal Microbiota. PLoS ONE.
   http://journals.plos.org/plosone/article?id=10.1371/journal.pone.0097500

3. Summa, K.C., Voigt, R.M., Forsyth, C.B., Shaikh, M., Cavanaugh, K. et al. Disruption of the Circadian Clock in Mice Increases Intestinal Permeability and Promotes Alcohol-Induced Hepatic Pathology and Inflammation. PLoS ONE (2013)
   http://journals.plos.org/plosone/article?id=10.1371/journal.pone.0067102

4. Helander, H.F. and Fändriks L. Surface area of the digestive tract – revisited. *Scandinavian Journal of Gastroenterology.* (2104)
   http://informahealthcare.com/doi/abs/10.3109/00365521.2014.898326

5. Net Carbohydrates – Wikipedia [Online]
   http://en.wikipedia.org/wiki/Net_carbohydrates

6. Potato Facts and Figures. International Potato Center.
   http://cipotato.org/potato/facts

7. FactFish – World: Tomatoes, production.
   http://www.factfish.com/statistic-country/world/tomatoes%2C%20production%20quantity

8. Isolauri, E., Majamaa, H., Arvola, T., Rantala, I., Virtanen, E., Arvilommi, H. Lactobacillus casei strain GG reverses increased intestinal permeability induced by cow milk in suckling rats.
   http://www.ncbi.nlm.nih.gov/pubmed/8253341

9. The Wine-o-scope (online).
   http://wineoscope.com/2011/11/16/189

10 Celiac disease: On the rise. (2010)
    http://www.mayo.edu/research/discoverys-edge/celiac-disease-rise

11 Fasano, A. and Catassi, C. Celiac Disease.
    http://www.nejm.org/doi/full/10.1056/NEJMcp1113994

12 2013 Survey – Consumer Attitudes About Nutrition. United Soybean Board.
    http://realfoodforager.com/7-reasons-to-avoid-soy-like-the-plague

13 Brandon, D.L., Bates, A.H., Friedman, M. ELISA analysis of soybean trypsin inhibitors in processed foods. (1991)
    http://www.ncbi.nlm.nih.gov/pubmed/1716818

14 Rackis, J. et al. The USDA trypsin inhibitor study. I. Background, objectives and procedural details, *Qualification of Plant Foods in Human Nutrition*, Vol. 35, 1985.

15 Jensen-Jarolim, E., Gajdzik, L., Habert, I., Kraft, D., Scheiner, O. and Graf, J. Spices Influence Permeability of Human Intestinal Epithelial Monolayers. (1998)

16 Sainio, E.-L., Jolanki, R., Hakala, E., & Kanerva, L. Metals and arsenic in eye shadows. *Contact Dermatitis*. (2001)
    http://www.ncbi.nlm.nih.gov/pubmed/10644018

17 Choi, A.L., Sun, G., Zhang, Y., Grandjean, P. Developmental fluoride neurotoxicity: A systematic review and meta-analysis. (2012)
    http://www.ncbi.nlm.nih.gov/pubmed/22820538

18 Centers for Disease Control and Prevention. 2012 CDC Water Fluoridation Statistics.
    http://www.cdc.gov/fluoridation/statistics/2012stats.htm

19 Moreira, M.A., André, L.C., Cardeal Zde L. Analysis of plasticiser migration to meat roasted in plastic bags by SPME-GC/MS.
    http://www.ncbi.nlm.nih.gov/pubmed/25704701

20 Bailey, M.T., Dowd, S. E. , Galley, J. D., Hufnagle, A.R., Allen,R.G., Lyte, M. Exposure to a social stressor alters the structure of the intestinal microbiota: Implications for stressor-induced immunomodulation.
    http://www.sciencedirect.com/science/article/pii/S0889159110005295

21 Blackburn, E. Part 3: Stress, Telomeres and Telomerase in Humans.
    https://www.youtube.com/watch?v=-INR1xZS5GY

22 Benson, H. And Klipper, M.Z. The Relaxation Response.

23 Relaxation techniques: Breath control helps quell errant stress response. (Online)
http://www.health.harvard.edu/mind-and-mood/relaxation-techniques-breath-control-helps-quell-errant-stress-response

24 Ghiya, S. and Lee, C.M. Influence of alternate nostril breathing on heart rate variability in non-practitioners of yogic breathing.
http://www.ncbi.nlm.nih.gov/pmc/articles/PMC3276936/

25 David, M. Eating Psychology and the Gut. Video presentation for the Healthy Gut Summit. (2015)

26 Vanessa Juth, V., Smyth, J.M. and Santuzzi, A.M. How Do You Feel? Self-esteem Predicts Affect, Stress, Social Interaction, and Symptom Severity during Daily Life in Patients with Chronic Illness.
http://www.ncbi.nlm.nih.gov/pmc/articles/PMC2996275/

27 Based on work by Melanie Fennell. Read her work in more detail here:
http://www.amazon.co.uk/Books-Melanie-Fennell/s?ie=UTF8&page=1&rh=n%3A266239%2Cp_27%3AMelanie Fennell

28 Capaldi, C.A., Dopko, R.L. and Zelenski, J.M. The relationship between nature connectedness and happiness: A meta-analysis. (2014)
http://journal.frontiersin.org/article/10.3389/fpsyg.2014.00976/abstract

29 Balseviciene,B., Sinkariova, L., Grazuleviciene, R., Andrusaityte, S., Uzdanaviciute, I,. Dedele, A. and Nieuwenhuijsen, M.J. Impact of Residential Greenness on Preschool Children's Emotional and Behavioral Problems.
http://www.mdpi.com/1660-4601/11/7/6757

30 Kuo, F.E. Parks and Other Green Environments: Essential Components of a Healthy Human Habitat.
http://www.nrpa.org/uploadedFiles/nrpa.org/Publications_and_Research/Research/Papers/MingKuo-Research-Paper.pdf

31 Chevalier, G., Sinatra, S.T., Oschman, J.L., Sokal, K. and Sokal, P. Earthing: Health Implications of Reconnecting the Human Body to the Earth's Surface.
http://www.hindawi.com/journals/jeph/2012/291541

APPENDIX

32 Ober, C.A. Grounding the human body to earth reduces chronic inflammation and related chronic pain. (2003)
http://www.esdjournal.com/articles/cober/earth.htm

33 Friis, R.H., Seaward, B.L, Dayer-Berenson, L. Managing Stress.

34 Light, K.C., Grewen, K.M., Amico, J.A. More frequent partner hugs and higher oxytocin levels are linked to lower blood pressure and heart rate in premenopausal women.
http://www.sciencedirect.com/science/article/pii/S0301051104001632

35 Martin, F-P.,J., Rezzi, S., Peré-Trepat, E., Kamlage, B., Collino, S., Leibold, E., Kastler, J., Rein, D., Fay, L.B. and Kochhar, S. Metabolic Effects of Dark Chocolate Consumption on Energy, Gut Microbiota, and Stress-Related Metabolism in Free-Living Subjects.
http://pubs.acs.org/doi/full/10.1021/pr900607v

36 Wirtz P.H., von Känel R., Meister R.E., et al. Dark chocolate intake buffers stress reactivity in humans. *J Am Coll Cardiol.* (2014)
http://content.onlinejacc.org/article.aspx?articleID=1851435

37 Sears, M.E., Kerr, K.J. and Bray, R.I. Arsenic, Cadmium, Lead, and Mercury in Sweat: A Systematic Review. (2012)
http://www.hindawi.com/journals/jeph/2012/184745

38 Clemes,S. Epidemiology of sedentary behaviour in office workers.
http://phirn.org.uk/files/2013/01/SClemes-Epidemiology-of-sedentary-behaviour-in-office-workers.pdf

39 Lalande, S., Okazaki, K., Yamazaki, T., Nose, H., Joyner, M.J., Johnson, B.D. Effects of interval walking on physical fitness in middle-aged individuals.
http://www.ncbi.nlm.nih.gov/pubmed/23804371

40 Centers for Disease Control and Prevention. Falls Among Older Adults: An Overview.
http://www.cdc.gov/HomeandRecreationalSafety/Falls/adultfalls.html

41 Franklin, B. *The Autobiography of Benjamin Franklin.*

42 The National Sleep Foundation. (2005)

43 Hirotsu, C., Rydlewski, M., Araújo, M.S., Tufik, S., Levy Andersen, M. Sleep Loss and Cytokines Levels in an Experimental Model of Psoriasis.
http://j.mp/1MWgcd4

44 Czeisler, C. A Sleep Epidemic. Tedx Cambridge.
    http://j.mp/1Cc9NXR

45 Hysing, M., Pallesen, S., Stormark, K.M., Jakobsen, R., Lundervold, A.J., Sivertsen, B. Sleep and use of electronic devices in adolescence: Results from a large population-based study.
    http://j.mp/1N1neeP

46 Czeisler, C.A., Shanahan, T.L., Klerman, E.B., Martens, H., Brotman, D.J., Emens, J.S, B.A., Klein, T. and Rizzo, J.F. Suppression of Melatonin Secretion in Some Blind Patients by Exposure to Bright Light.
    http://www.ncbi.nlm.nih.gov/pubmed/7990870

47 Ohayon, M.M. Nocturnal awakenings and comorbid disorders in the American general population. (2006)
    http://j.mp/1MWgcd4

48 Haixia Qin,H., Zheng,X., Zhong,X., Shetty,A.K., Elias,P.M. and Bollag, W.B. Aquaporin-3 in Keratinocytes and Skin: Its Role and Interaction with Phospholipase D2.
    http://www.ncbi.nlm.nih.gov/pmc/articles/PMC3061340/

49 Breternitz, M., Kowatzki, D., Langenauer, M., Elsner, P., Fluhr, J.W. Placebo-controlled, double-blind, randomized, prospective study of a glycerol-based emollient on eczematous skin in atopic dermatitis: biophysical and clinical evaluation.
    http://www.ncbi.nlm.nih.gov/pubmed/18025807

50 Zuckerbraun, H.L., Babich, H., May, R., Sinensky, M.C. Triclosan: cytotoxicity, mode of action, and induction of apoptosis in human gingival cells in vitro.
    http://www.ncbi.nlm.nih.gov/pubmed/9584909?dopt=Abstract

51 Standard Badminton Court Layout.
    http://www.badminton-information.com/badminton-court.html

52 Herculano-Houzel, S. and Lent, R. Isotropic Fractionator: A Simple, Rapid Method for the Quantification of Total Cell and Neuron Numbers in the Brain.
    http://www.jneurosci.org/content/25/10/2518.full

53 Corcoran, C.D., Thomas, P., Phillips, J., O'Keane, V. Vagus nerve stimulation in chronic treatment-resistant depression: Preliminary findings of an open-label study.
    http://bjp.rcpsych.org/content/189/3/282.full

54 That gut feeling. American Psychological Association.
http://www.apa.org/monitor/2012/09/gut-feeling.aspx

55 Mayer, E.A. Gut feelings: The emerging biology of gut–brain communication. *Nat Rev Neurosci.* (2011)
http://www.ncbi.nlm.nih.gov/pmc/articles/PMC3845678/

56 Bornstein, J.C. Serotonin in the Gut: What Does It Do?
http://www.ncbi.nlm.nih.gov/pmc/articles/PMC3272651/

57 Yadav, V.K., Balaji, S., Suresh, P.S., Sherry Liu,X., Lu,X., Li, Z., Guo, X.E., Mann, J.J., Balapure, A.K., Gershon, M.D., Medhamurthy, R., Vidal, M., Karsenty, G.& Ducy, P. Pharmacological inhibition of gut-derived serotonin synthesis is a potential bone anabolic treatment for osteoporosis.
http://www.nature.com/nm/journal/v16/n3/abs/nm.2098.html

58 Major Crops Grown in the United States.
http://www.epa.gov/agriculture/ag101/cropmajor.html

59 Diamond, J. The worst mistake in the history of the human race. *Discover Magazine*, University of California at Los Angeles, Medical School.

60 Lenoir, M., Serre, F., Cantin, L. and Ahmed, S.H. Intense sweetness surpasses cocaine reward. (2007)
http://journals.plos.org/plosone/article?id=10.1371/journal.pone.0000698

61 McDonald's Burger Looks the Same – 14 Years Later.
http://newsfeed.time.com/2013/04/25/mcdonalds-burger-looks-the-same-14-years-later/

62 van der Hulst, R.R, von Meyenfeldt, M.F., Soeters, P.B. Glutamine: An essential amino acid for the gut. *Nutrition.* (1996)
http://www.ncbi.nlm.nih.gov/pubmed/8974125

63 Ban, K. and Kozar, R.A. Glutamine protects against apoptosis via downregulation of Sp3 in intestinal epithelial cells.
http://www.ncbi.nlm.nih.gov/pubmed/20884886

64 Larson, S.D., Li, J., Chung, D.H.and Evers, B.M. Molecular Mechanisms Contributing to Glutamine-Mediated Intestinal Cell Survival.
http://www.ncbi.nlm.nih.gov/pmc/articles/PMC2432018/

65. Forrest, K.Y. and Stuhldreher, W.L. Prevalence and correlates of vitamin D deficiency in US adults. Department of Public Health and Social Work, Slippery Rock University of Pennsylvania. (2011)
http://1.usa.gov/18b4etq

66. Reid, G. The Scientific Basis for Probiotic Strains of Lactobacillus.
http://aem.asm.org/content/65/9/3763

67. Picard, C., Fioramonti, J., Francois, A., Robinson, T., Neant, F., Matuchansky, C. Review article: Bifidobacteria as probiotic agents – physiological effects and clinical benefits.
http://www.ncbi.nlm.nih.gov/pubmed/16167966

68. Patel, R.M., Wei Denning, P. Therapeutic Use of Prebiotics, Probiotics, and Postbiotics to Prevent Necrotizing Enterocolitis: What is the Current Evidence?
http://www.ncbi.nlm.nih.gov/pmc/articles/PMC3575601/

69. Cieslinska, A., Kaminski, S.T., Kostyra, E., Sienkiewicz-Szłapka, E. Beta-casomorphin 7 in raw and hydrolyzed milk derived from cows of alternative β-casein genotypes.
http://www.academia.edu/1368959/Beta-casomorphin_7_in_raw_and_hydrolyzed_milk_derived_from_cows_of_alternative_%CE%B2-casein_genotypes

70. European Food Safety Authority. Review of the potential health impact of β-casomorphins and related peptides.
http://www.efsa.europa.eu/en/scdocs/doc/231r.pdf

71. European Food Safety Authority. Crop Production by Country.
http://faostat3.fao.org/browse/Q/*/E

72. Diamond, J. The worst mistake in the history of the human race. *Discover Magazine*, University of California at Los Angeles, Medical School.

73. Phytic acid.
http://en.wikipedia.org/wiki/Phytic_acid

74. World Market of Sugar and Sweeteners.
https://www.uni-hohenheim.de/fileadmin/einrichtungen/stevia/downloads/World_Market_Sugar.pdf

75 International Sugar Organization. Alternative Sweeteners in a High Sugar Price Environment. (2012)
    http://www.isosugar.org

76 Yang, Q. Gain weight by 'going diet?' Artificial sweeteners and the neurobiology of sugar cravings. *Neuroscience*. (2010)
    http://www.ncbi.nlm.nih.gov/pmc/articles/PMC2892765/

77 Cong, W., Cohen, S. Article: Artificial Sweeteners and Leptin; Impaired Lipid Storage and Starvation.
    http://irp.nih.gov/catalyst/v22i3/artificial-and-leptin-impaired-lipid-storage-and-starvation

78 Suez, J., Korem, T., Zeevi, D., Zilberman-Schapira, G., Thaiss, C.A., Maza, O., Israeli, D., Zmora, N., Gilad, S., Weinberger, A., Kuperman, Y., Harmelin,A., Kolodkin-Gal, I., Shapiro, H., Halpern, Z., Segal, E. and Elinav, E. Artificial sweeteners induce glucose intolerance by altering the gut microbiota.
    http://www.nature.com/nature/journal/v514/n7521/full/nature13793.html

79 Gavura, S. Article: Fatigued by a Fake Disease.
    https://www.sciencebasedmedicine.org/fatigued-by-a-fake-disease/

80 Gordon, I., Vander Wyk, B.C., Bennetta, R.H., Cordeaux, C., Lucasa, M.V., Eilbott, J.A., Zagoory-Sharon, O., Leckmand, J.F., Feldman, R., Pelphreya, K.A. Oxytocin enhances brain function in children with autism.
    http://www.pnas.org/content/110/52/20953.abstract

81 Brandt, C. and Pedersen, B.K. The Role of Exercise-Induced Myokines in Muscle Homeostasis and the Defense against Chronic Diseases.
    http://www.hindawi.com/journals/bmri/2010/520258/

82 So, B., Kim, H-J., Kim, J., Song, W. Exercise-induced myokines in health and metabolic diseases.
    http://www.sciencedirect.com/science/article/pii/S2213422014000705

83 Biological Clock Human. Yassine Mrabet fixed by Addicted04
    [GFDL (http://www.gnu.org/copyleft/fdl.html) or CC BY-SA 3.0 (http://creativecommons.org/licenses/by-sa/3.0)], via Wikimedia Commons

84 Smolensky, M., Lamberg, L. The Body Clock Guide to Better Health: How to Use your Body's Natural Clock to Fight Illness and Achieve Maximum Health. (2001)

85 Bissonnette, R. Psoriasis: Why Does it Come With a Greater Risk of Heart Attack and Stroke?
http://www.medscape.com/viewarticle/772802

86 Chang, E.Y., Hammerberg, C., Fisher, G., Baadsgaard, O., Ellis, C.N., Voorhees, J.J., Cooper, K.D. T-cell activation is potentiated by cytokines released by lesional psoriatic, but not normal, epidermis. http://www.ncbi.nlm.nih.gov/pubmed/1359841

87 Fry, L., Baker, B.S., Powles, A.V. and Engstrand, L. Psoriasis is not an autoimmune disease?
http://onlinelibrary.wiley.com/doi/10.1111/exd.12572/full

88 Salahuddin, T., Natarajan, N., Selwaness, M., Sadek, A., Playford, M., Doveikis, J., Nanda, N., Bluemke, D., Mehta, N. Vascular inflammation in the aorta is related to coronary plaque burden in psoriasis.
http://content.onlinejacc.org/article.aspx?articleid=2199102

89 Ahlehoff, O., Gislason, O.H., Charlot, M., Jørgensen, C.H., Lindhardsen, L., Bjerring Olesen, J., Abildstrøm, S.Z., Skov, L., Torp-Pedersen, C., Hansen, P.R. Psoriasis is associated with clinically significant cardiovascular risk: A Danish nationwide cohort study.
http://forskning.ku.dk/find-en-forsker/?pure=da%2Fpublications%2Fpsoriasis-is-associated-with-clinically-significant-cardiovascular-risk-a-danish-nationwide-cohort-study%285556b970-b45b-4556-9bd8-3cbc825d1c67%29.html

90 Plengvidhya, V., Breidt,F., Lu, Z. and Fleming, H.P. DNA Fingerprinting of Lactic Acid Bacteria in Sauerkraut Fermentations.
http://www.ncbi.nlm.nih.gov/pubmed/23102182

91 Ng, S.W., Slining, M.M., Popkin, B.M. Use of caloric and noncaloric sweeteners in US consumer packaged foods, 2005-2009.
http://www.ncbi.nlm.nih.gov/pmc/articles/PMC2168044/

92 Lewis, S. J. and Heaton, K.W. Stool Form Scale as a Useful Guide to Intestinal Transit Time.
http://informahealthcare.com/doi/abs/10.3109/00365529709011203

93 Riegler, G., Esposito, I. Bristol scale stool form. A still valid help in medical practice and clinical research. (2001)
http://www.ncbi.nlm.nih.gov/pubmed/11875684

94 Zimmaro, Bliss D., Larson S.J., Burr J.K., Savik K. Reliability of a stool consistency classification system.
http://www.ncbi.nlm.nih.gov/pubmed/11707763

Readings

In addition to trawling through hundreds of medical journal articles, here are some of the books I read while writing this book.

Books are listed in no particular order.
- *The Primal Connection* by Mark Sisson
- *The Paleo Approach* by Sarah Ballantyne
- *The Paleo Diet for Athletes* by Loren Cordain and Joe Friel
- *Primal Body, Primal Mind* by Nora T. Gedgaudas
- *The Hormone Cure* by Sara Gottfried
- *Healing Psoriasis* by John O. A. Pagano
- *The Science of Leaky Gut Syndrome* by Case Adams
- *Sweat Therapy* by Stephen A. Colmant
- *An Introduction to Coping with Low Self-Esteem* by Melanie Fennell and Lee Brosan

APPENDIX

About the author and other books

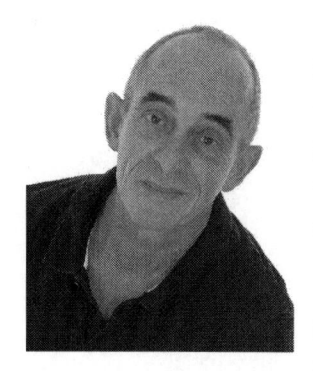

Howard Rybko was born in Johannesburg, South Africa, in 1956. He graduated as an MD from the University Of Witwatersrand Medical School in 1981. He worked in research for two years and then in private medical practice, where he specialized in diet and weight management.

Sometime in the late 80s he started working with medical software. He has been involved in sports nutrition and performance since 1992, specializing in cycling.

Review request

Please consider writing a review of The Four Horsemen of Psoriasis, I would love to hear your feedback. Enter this link to go to your reviews page on Amazon: http://j.mp/1IJDgLa

Upcoming book

I am currently working on a new book on health aging that will extend established concepts in the low-carb and Paleo diets to include pieces of the puzzle that are missing from a completely healthy lifestyle.

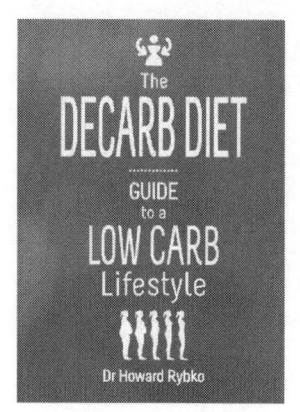

Other books

The Decarb Diet: Guide to a Low Carb Lifestyle – published in 2013